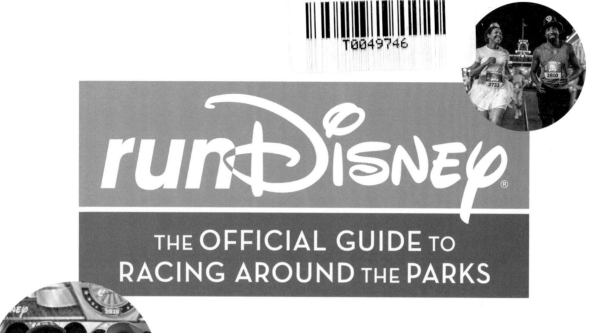

runDisney®

THE OFFICIAL GUIDE TO RACING AROUND THE PARKS

SCOTT DOUGLAS

FOREWORD BY **JEFF GALLOWAY**
SELECT SIDEBARS BY **JEFF GALLOWAY**
AND **MOLLY HUDDLE**

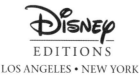

DISNEP

EDITIONS

LOS ANGELES • NEW YORK

CONTENTS

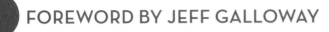

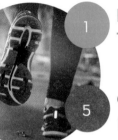

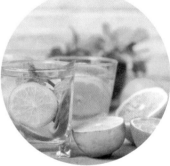

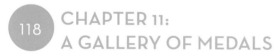

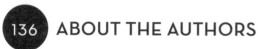
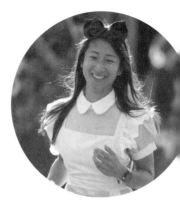

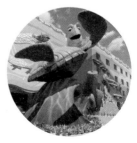

All photographs copyright © Disney Enterprises, Inc., except the following:
Photographs on back cover, and pages ii, 7, 13, 16, 18, 22, 32, 33, 36, 39, 41, 42, 44, 45, 46, 49, 51, 54, 56, 57, 58, 59, 60, 61, 62, 63, 67, 68, 69, 71, 82, 85, 94, 95, 109: Courtesy of Purestock © PureStock/SuperStock
Author photograph of Jeff Galloway: Courtesy of Daniel Menacher
Author photograph of Molly Huddle: Courtesy of Matthew Caputo
Author photograph of Scott Douglas: Courtesy of Stacey Cramp

The following are copyrights or trademarks of their respective owners: *Disney Cruise Line*® Ships; *Disney Dream*® Cruise Ship; *Disney Springs*™; *Disney Village*®; Disney's All-Star Movies Resort; Disney's All-Star Music Resort; Disney's All-Star Sports Resort; *Disney's Animal Kingdom*® Lodge; *Disney's Animal Kingdom*® Theme Park; *Disney's Animal Kingdom*® Villas—Kidani Village; Disney's Art of Animation Resort; Disney's Beach Club Resort and Villas; Disney's BoardWalk Inn and Villas; Disney's Caribbean Beach Resort; Disney's Contemporary Resort; Disney's Coronado Springs Resort; Disney's Fort Wilderness Resort; Disney's Grand Floridian Resort & Spa; *Disney's Hollywood Studios*®; Disney's Old Key West Resort; Disney's Polynesian Resort; Disney's Pop Century Resort; Disney's Port Orleans Resort—French Quarter; Disney's Port Orleans Resort—Riverside; Disney's Saratoga Springs Resort & Spa; *Disney's Sequoia Lodge*®; Disney's Wilderness Lodge; Disney's Yacht Club Resort; EPCOT®; *Fantasyland*® Area; *Frontierland*® Area; "it's a small world," *It's A Small World*® Attraction; *Magic Kingdom*® Park; *Main Street, U.S.A.*® Area; *Space Mountain*® Attraction; *Splash Mountain*® Attraction; *Tomorrowland*® Area; *Walt Disney Studios*® Park; *Walt Disney World*® Resort; and World Showcase.

Corkcicle® is a Registered Trademark of Corkcicle, LLC. All rights reserved.

ISBN 978-1-368-05496-6
FAC-029261-23313
Library of Congress Control Number: 2020937581

First Paperback Edition, March 2024   10 9 8 7 6 5 4 3 2 1

Printed in the United States of America

The recommendations in this book are not intended to replace or conflict with the advice given to you by your physician or other health professionals. All matters regarding your health require medical supervision. Consult your physician before adopting the suggestions in this book. Before using any vitamins mentioned in this book, be sure to consult with the appropriate medical authorities and check the product's label for any warnings or caution. Pregnant women are advised that special precautions may pertain to any exercise program they undertake. If you are pregnant, talk to your doctor before undertaking any exercises suggested in this book. The author and publisher disclaim any liability directly or indirectly from the use of the material in this book by any person.

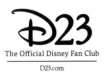

The Official Disney Fan Club
D23.com

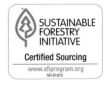

FOREWORD

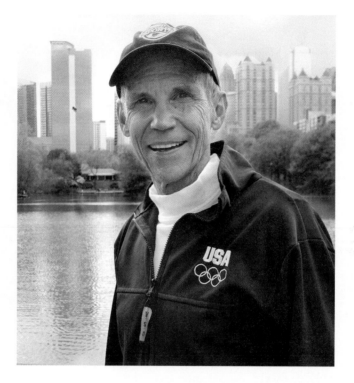

What would motivate you to travel to a race? How about an upbeat and fun weekend in which all family members or companions can participate? The runDisney events are known for their great organization, and for always being staged in a safe and supportive environment (with convenient transportation, restaurants, and entertainment from morning to night). If you want to be entertained, runDisney does it best!

I'm proud to have designed the highly successful runDisney training schedules for participants at all levels and for all abilities. Hundreds of thousands have moved off the couch and finished 5Ks, 10Ks, half marathons—and even marathons . . . and have done it willingly—even with a smile.

The best part about being the official training consultant for runDisney is hearing from over ten thousand runners and walkers each year. Many credit the runDisney training journey for changing their lives. I hear again and again from participants about their dramatic weight loss, how they've decided to pursue new careers, breakthroughs in dealing with personal stress, and regaining control and balance.

You'll have your best runDisney experience if you come to the weekend event fit, injury-free, and ready to take in all the fun. And that's where this book comes in: it's full of common sense advice and insider info on running in general and runDisney in particular. I hope you'll read it carefully.

Join me and find your runDisney magic. Come by my booth at the race expo. I want to hear your story.

—Jeff Galloway,
Olympian and official runDisney training consultant

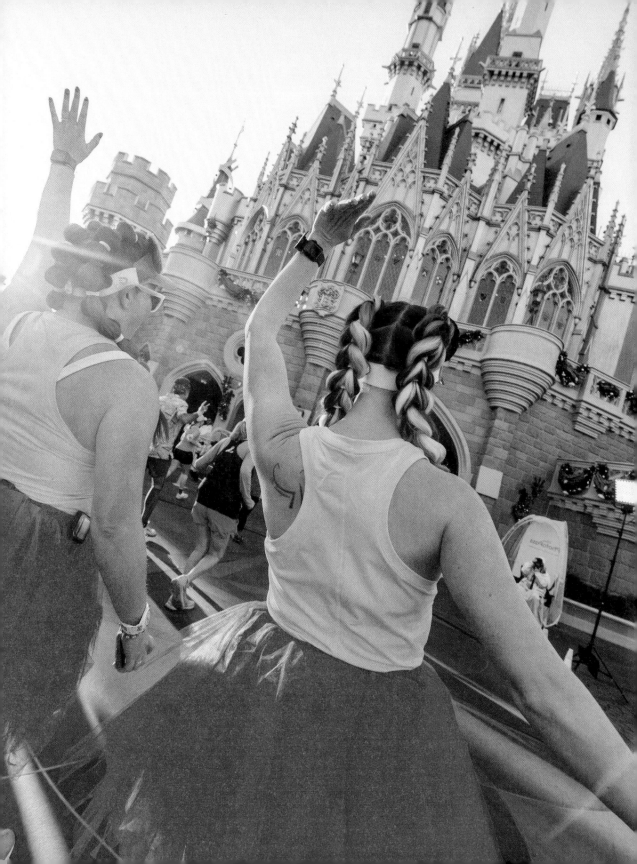

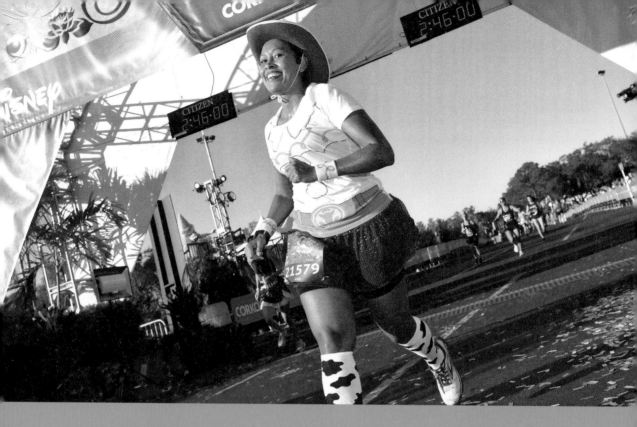

INTRODUCTION:
THE JOYS AND BENEFITS OF RUNNING

Running is amazing. Millions of runners around the world can't imagine their lives without it. And for good reason—no other activity is so accessible and convenient, while improving your physical and mental health and your quality of life.

In this book, we'll mostly look at the "how" aspect of running. You'll learn *how* to get going if you're not yet a runner, *how* to improve your speed and endurance, *how* to eat and dress like a runner, and *how* to avoid running injuries. In the second half of the book, we'll dive into the magical world of runDisney, one of the most fun experiences you'll ever have.

First, though, let's briefly get into the "why" aspect of running. What motivates millions to regularly do this thing that, on the face of it, might seem more trouble than it's worth?

For starters, there are the physical and mental health benefits. These benefits are often what initially attracts people to running. Everyone knows in some vague sense that running is good for you. But just how good? Here's a little detail.

COMPARED TO SEDENTARY PEOPLE

- Runners have lower rates of several chronic conditions, including heart disease, high blood pressure, high cholesterol, and diabetes.

- Runners have lower rates of some forms of cancer, including breast, prostate, kidney, and colon.

- Runners have fewer strokes.

- Runners are more likely to be at a healthy weight.

- Runners are less likely to suffer from moderate to severe depression and anxiety.

- Runners are more likely to score higher on tests of cognitive ability, and less likely to experience cognitive decline with age.

- Runners are less likely to develop osteoarthritis. (Yes, you read that correctly. Details in chapter 5.)

- Runners are less likely to develop osteoporosis.

And if all that isn't enough, in a given time period, runners are less likely to die.

What a list! Even better is that it doesn't take tons of running to get these benefits. As little as ten to fifteen miles a week will significantly improve your health on these fronts and other ways. (There's even evidence that runners are less likely than sedentary people to develop cataracts.) A few short runs per week are a small investment for such huge payoffs.

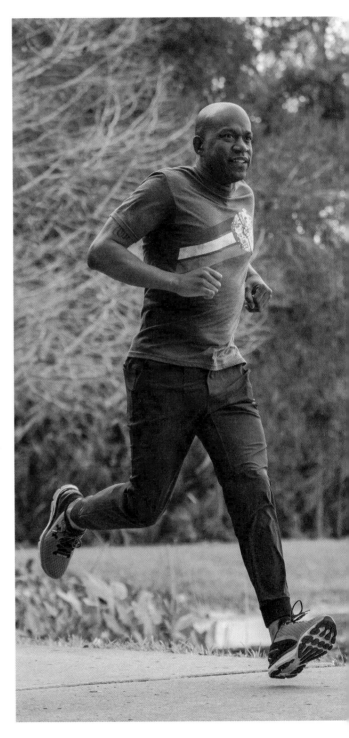

RUN FOR FUN

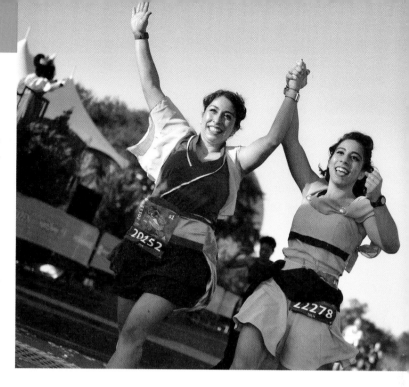

The thing is, once runners have established some baseline fitness and a regular running schedule, many are motivated to move beyond just maintaining these worthy benefits. They come to think of running not as something they "should" do, but something they *want* to do. They would run for the rest of their lives even if doing so didn't improve their health.

Why? Because running is fun. That's right, *fun*. "Fun" doesn't just mean activities where you're constantly laughing and smiling. (Although if you pay attention, you'll notice there's no truth to the old claim—often uttered by those who don't run—that "I never see runners smile.")

What's *fun* is anything you do that improves your quality of life. You might not always be smiling while listening to your favorite music, playing with your children, pursuing a hobby, or sitting quietly next to your partner, but you know your life would be poorer without those regular experiences.

Fun is built into the very DNA of running. There's the sense of accomplishment, socializing, quality solo time, adventure, exploration, play, challenge, reward, encounters with nature, working toward achieving a goal, living in the moment, mental clarity, a state of flow, and so much more during a typical week of running.

Organized races enhance and add a whole other level of fun to your running experiences. You don't need to do races to have fun as a runner, but you're guaranteed to have even *more* fun if you do. Races add subtle quality-of-life aspects of fun; there's the satisfaction of having challenged yourself, plus the more straightforward elements of fun mentioned earlier. You're unlikely to see more smiles and cheering than at a road race.

That's particularly true at a runDisney event, where whimsy and work combine to produce something magical. Where else can you have world-class entertainment, with some of the world's most beloved characters cheering you on, as you run through treasured theme parks?

On top of all that, every runDisney event has a special theme that adds even more fun (if that's possible) to the weekend. At most races, costumed runners are the exception, but when you participate in a runDisney event, you'll be surrounded by them! They're your fellow Disney fans! You'll be spending time with them whether you're running a race or supporting someone who is! Why? You're at one of the world's top travel destinations for goodness' sake, and whoever joins in is guaranteed to have at least as good a time as you.

runDisney is an experience you can't get or duplicate anywhere else. If that's not fun, then what is?

ABOUT THIS BOOK

The two most important words in running could be these: "It depends." In running, it's said, "we're all an experiment of one." The training program, shoes, and diet that work well for you might not be best for your best running friend. They might not even be the best training program, shoes, and diet for you a year from now. All of us come to running as unique, ever-changing—and evolving—individuals. Beware of anyone giving running advice in a universal, one-size-fits-all manner.

That said, there are basic principles and best practices that apply to almost all runners. Various ways of succeeding and achieving as a runner have been worked out by the tens of millions of runners who have paved the way for you. It's quite likely that what these runners have discovered to be the best approach will also work well for you. Outliers are, by definition, the exceptions.

The advice in this book comes from three lifelong runners with more than a combined century of experience in the sport. Two of the three are Olympians; the other is a veteran running journalist. You can be confident in the guidance you'll get on how to run farther and faster, how to maintain motivation, what to eat and wear, and how to fully enjoy all that running has to offer. The guidance comes from those who have immersed themselves in all aspects of running, from the highest competitive levels to regular contact with those just taking their first steps . . . and are venturing into a new sport/lifestyle.

That insider's knowledge extends to the second half of the book, where we'll look at how to have the best possible runDisney experience.

So, if you're ready to have some fun, let's get going, shall we?

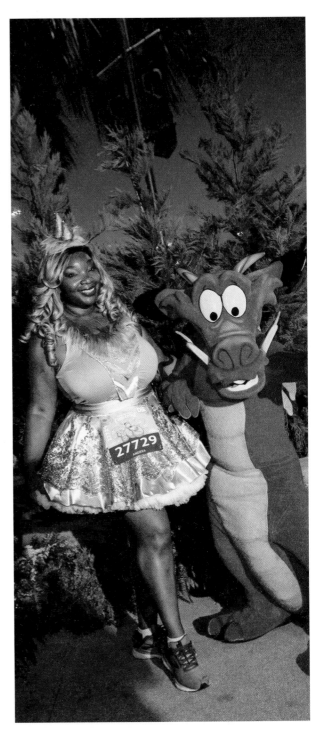

CHAPTER 1:
HOW TO START RUNNING

Every runner was a *beginning runner* at some point. Even those runners who seem to float down your street were newbies once. They, too, sometimes got out of breath, hurt all over, lacked motivation, and wondered just what is supposedly so great about this running thing.

They and millions of others stuck with it, and now can't imagine their lives without running. You can join them. You've already taken the most important step, even if you haven't yet run a step. You've decided to become a runner. That commitment sets you up for a lifetime of health and fitness, fun and friendship, and accomplishment and satisfaction.

Now it's time to turn that commitment into reality. In this chapter, we'll look at how to get going as a runner—how fast, how far . . . basics like that. We'll also explore ways to increase your chances of success and overcome some of the common challenges new runners face.

You'll want to read this chapter even if you're not a new runner. There's lots of hard-earned wisdom on how to succeed over the long-term as a runner.

HOW FAST TO RUN

Slow down!

Seriously, slow down. One of the main reasons that new runners find running challenging is that they haven't yet learned how to pace themselves. Many start off strong on a typical run, but then soon after are gasping for breath. They slow dramatically, maybe walk or stop to catch their breath. The rest of the run for them after that initial flash of speed and can-do spirit is miserable. They think, "Running sucks."

Misconceptions about what running should feel like—and how one should feel when doing it—magnify this problem. Maybe you think it's supposed to hurt, so if you're under duress right from the get-go you must be doing it right.

But that's not how it works. Even the best runners in the world do the overwhelming majority of their runs at a conversational pace. They can talk in complete sentences at any time. The reason? They're running at a relaxed pace, with minimal effort (from their perspective). They start their runs slowly, allowing their bodies to warm up, and increase the pace only as doing so feels comfortable. You will never see these runners going faster one minute into their run than they are going halfway through their workout.

So, again, slow down. Think in terms of effort, not pace. Start at a light effort. Yes, your breathing will increase rapidly in the first few minutes. Just keep it under control by not asking more of your body than what it's currently primed for. If you start in this gentle way, your pace will naturally pick up, even though your effort level will remain the same.

Aim to maintain this gentle effort level on all of your runs for at least your first month. Don't worry about pace. Just cover the ground at whatever speed allows you to be able to speak in complete sentences.

You might find that, no matter how slow you go, you can't maintain that conversational effort level without stopping to walk. That's totally fine. Mixing walking and running is a time-honored way to cover all sorts of distances. Some runners start with a run-walk program and eventually shift to all running. Others find that they enjoy the mix more than straight running even when they're capable of covering a given distance without walking. It's all good!

For more on how to mix running and walking into your routine, see "The Galloway Run-Walk-Run Method" sidebar later in the book.

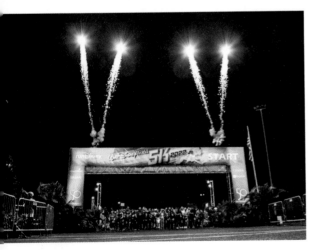

HOW FAR TO RUN

There's no minimum mileage you have to cover for a run to "count." Whatever you can do, great. Stay at around that amount for several runs until you can honestly say it doesn't feel like you've done enough. In the next chapter, we'll look in detail at how best to increase your mileage safely.

Starting out, err on the side of caution. As we'll see in chapter 5, a leading cause of injury is running more than you're currently able to handle structurally. Experienced runners don't head out every time to go as far as they can. Most of them are capable of running three or four times as far as what they cover on a typical run.

At some point you'll probably want to start pushing the envelope, to see if you can gradually increase the distance of your standard run. Those excursions should be rare, a few times a month at most. You want to finish most runs feeling like you could have kept going without feeling significantly more fatigued if you had to.

HOW OFTEN TO RUN

Two or three times a week is a good goal starting out. You're still a runner if you run less frequently than that. But two or three runs a week will have a multiplier effect that won't kick in if you run more sporadically. Your fitness level will build much more quickly, which will then make the following week's runs more doable. Your fitness will increase that much more, and success will build on success.

Going two or three times a week will also help you find your rhythm as a runner. Each run won't feel like you're starting from scratch, either physically or logistically. Establishing that more frequent

routine will make running seem like a normal, regular part of your life rather than something that happens only when your schedule is wide open.

Hold off on going more than three times a week until you string together a month or two of consistent running. Then add another day per week if you want to. This gradual approach is especially important if you're coming to running from having been sedentary for a while. First, establish a good base. Then you'll have the rest of your life to build on it.

WHERE TO RUN

Running is rightfully praised for its convenience. Unlike most other sports, you can be a runner pretty much anywhere. So, the ultimate answer to the query "Where to run?" is "wherever in the world you find yourself."

In your everyday life, that will probably mean running around your neighborhood. Running on the roads is convenient and more mentally stimulating than running around a track or on a treadmill. Run against traffic so that you can see what drivers are up to. Try to find roads that aren't too busy and that don't have huge cambers toward the sides, which is where you'll usually be running to avoid vehicles. Regularly running on slanted roads can throw your hips out of whack and set you up for injury.

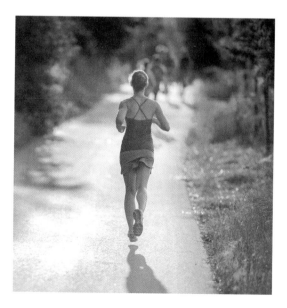

THE GALLOWAY RUN-WALK-RUN METHOD

 After running almost every day for over sixty years, I continue to enjoy every run and feel great afterward because of my strategic run-walk-run (RWR) method from the outset of each run. RWR works well for all runners, but is especially useful in your early days as a runner. This method is the basis for all of my official runDisney training programs. Here's how it works—and some of the benefits:

- RWR gives you cognitive and physical control over each workout.
- The right strategy eliminates exhaustion and allows you to carry on all of your life activities, even after long events such as marathons.
- RWR motivates beginners to get off the couch and run—and can help eliminate injury.
- Veteran runners who became burned-out or injured are making a comeback by following my RWR steps.
- RWR produces faster times in races (on average, more than seven minutes faster when followed in a half marathon run for example).
- Adjusting to the right RWR workout can make every run enjoyable.
- Runners who use the right RWR approach get all of the benefits of running without pain or injury.

WALK BEFORE YOU GET TIRED: The RWR method is very simple: you run for a short segment, take a walk break, and keep repeating this pattern.

Most of us, even when untrained, can walk for several miles before fatigue sets in, because we're genetically designed to walk efficiently for hours. Running is more work, because you have to lift your body off the ground and then absorb the shock of the landing . . . over and over. This is why those who run continuously will exhaust the calf muscle and irritate their "weak links" much sooner. Each walk break from the outset can erase fatigue buildup, and reduce the stress buildup on weak links.

USE A SHORT, GENTLE WALKING STRIDE: Walk gently with a relatively short stride to reduce orthopedic stress. If you want to practice a faster walk-pace, work on improved cadence.

NO NEED TO ELIMINATE WALK BREAKS AS YOU GET FITTER: Don't assume that you need to reduce walk breaks as your fitness improves. Most of my runners find that small adjustments in their RWR strategies actually lead to faster times. Those who increase the running segment and walk less tend to have slower times, more aches and pains, and a longer recovery period. As you

Sidewalks remove the danger of vehicles, though they often may present their own challenges. Footing can be tricky—due to the ups and downs of uneven walkways, as well as curbs and driveways. Drivers emerging from cross streets and driveways are less likely to see you than if you were running on the road. Plus, lots of other people also use sidewalks, so you might find yourself repeatedly dashing out into the road to get around them.

adjust the running and the walking on each run, you gain control over how you feel—which is empowering in itself.

RWR activates your conscious brain, which can keep the ancient subconscious brain from triggering negative hormones as you experience fatigue and other stresses. If a given strategy is too tough, activate the conscious brain by changing the run-walk-run segments.

The best way to stay with your strategy (and stick to the time segments you think work best for you) is to use a timer. It can be set up for any two intervals; an audible beep tells you when to resume a run, and when to break for a walk—plus tracks the time you have set for each period. These timers are available at *JeffGalloway.com* and at my booth at the runDisney expos.

THE RIGHT RUN-WALK-RUN MIX

After having heard from more than half a million runners who have used the RWR method at various paces, I've analyzed and tabulated the strategies based upon the most successful by pace per mile.

Reports from thousands of runners who have used variations between twenty seconds and sixty seconds tend to show that most receive as much recovery from a twenty- to thirty-second walk break as from a longer walk. In fact, there's usually a slowdown during the second half of a one-minute walk break. This makes it harder to start running again toward the end of a long run or race. By shortening both the run segment and the walk segment, fatigue at the end of the run can be reduced significantly.

—Jeff Galloway, Olympian and official runDisney training consultant

RUN-WALK-RUN STRATEGIES

Pace/mile	Run	Walk
7:00	6 minutes	30 seconds (or run a mile/walk 40 seconds)
7:30	5 minutes	30 seconds (or 2:30/:15)
8:00	4 minutes	30 seconds (or 2:00/:15)
8:30	3 minutes	30 seconds (or 2:00/:20)
9:00	2 minutes	30 seconds (or 1:20/:20)
9:30–10:45	1:30/:30 or 1:00/:20 or :45/:15 or 1:00/:30 or :40/:20	
10:45–12:15	1:00/:30 or :40/:20 or :30/:15 or :30/:30 or :20/:20	
12:15–14:15	:30/:30 or :20/:20 or :15/:15	
14:15–15:45	:15/:30	
15:45–17:00	:10/:30 or :57/:30	
17:00–18:30	:8/:30 or :5/:25 or :10/:30	
18:30–20:00	:5/:30 or :5/:25 or :4/:30	

Recreational paths are a blessing if you have easy access to them. It's worth seeking out these vehicle-free alternatives for the chance to more easily get in a nice carefree running rhythm.

Running on trails has its own magical qualities.

"Green exercise," or working out in nature, is increasingly proven to provide more tranquility and other positive emotions than doing the same exercise elsewhere. Time seems to take on a different quality when you're running in a forest or

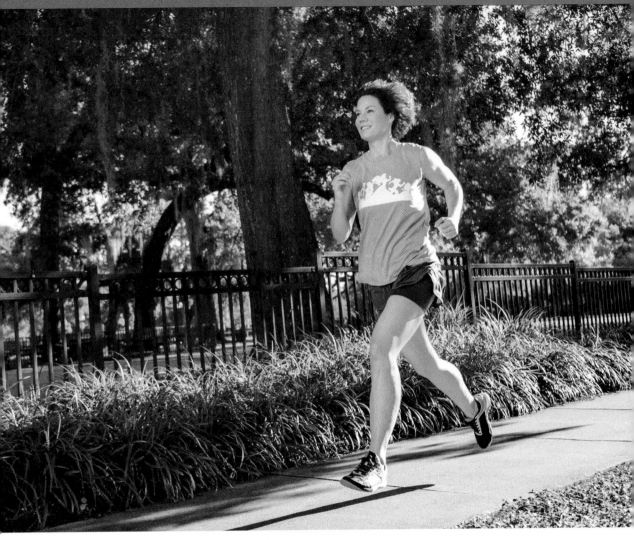

alongside a mountain. Twenty minutes might fly by when running in a natural setting, while that same twenty minutes running in a crowded urban setting can feel more like a slog. Trails and other softer surfaces also offer another benefit: they're naturally cushioned, reducing some of the impactful forces you endure when navigating streets of asphalt or cement sidewalks.

Finally, there's the treadmill. There's nothing wrong with being a runner who frequently hits the treadmill. It's a safe, reliable environment that you have complete control over. You can stop whenever you want, and it doesn't matter what the weather is. Treadmills also ostensibly provide a softer surface to land on than asphalt or sidewalks. Still, once you've established a good running routine, see whether or not you enjoy running more outdoors. There's a whole world out there to see! If you're planning to do a runDisney event (or another race), you'll definitely want to leave the treadmill and head outside for key practice runs. Otherwise, running on a stationary surface will feel weird enough to detract from your performance and enjoyment.

HOW TO INCREASE YOUR CHANCES OF SUCCESS

Use these tips to find meaning and pleasure in your runs, and therefore be more likely to stick with it.

SET THE RIGHT KIND OF GOALS: Humans are wired to be goal-oriented. Probably everything worthwhile you've achieved resulted from you telling yourself, *I want to do X*, and then working methodically toward meeting that goal.

You might think, "I have enough pressure in my life. I don't want my running to be one more thing that feels like work." But think about it: You've decided to be a runner. Right there you've set a goal. That doesn't automatically make running a chore. It means you've decided your life will be better if you're a runner.

You'll go far toward meeting that overall goal if you have more specific shorter-term goals. The qualities of good goals are:

- **They're personally meaningful:** Set running goals that speak to your dreams and desires, not someone else's. You should be able to imagine how happy and satisfied you'll be when you meet your goals. If you can't conjure those mental images (or envision them being within reach), the goal probably isn't that meaningful to you. The right goals will ignite the fire and motivate you to keep working during momentary lags that are bound to arise.

- **They're ambitious:** Good goals will make you stretch (figuratively, not literally, although literal stretching may well help you meet your running goals). If you can currently run one mile without stopping, setting as a key goal of running one and a half miles without stopping is probably underselling yourself—and your full potential. Think of goals that will require regular commitment, but will result in significant advancement in some way.

- **They're realistic:** There's a difference between ambitious and crazy. If you can currently run one mile without stopping, setting the goal of running ten miles without stopping by the end of the following week isn't going to end well. A good goal is reasonably within your grasp if you do the work.

- **They're specific:** Good goals are quantifiable in two ways: they provide a yes-or-no way of knowing whether you've achieved them, and they happen within a specific time period. The goal *I want to get in better shape* is too vague. How much better? By when? Goals that are too open-ended won't motivate you to regularly work toward them. In contrast, the goal of *wanting to run three miles without stopping by the end of next month* gives you a quantifiable measure of success and impetus to keep chipping away at drawing closer to the objective—and accomplishing it.

- **They're stepping-stones:** A good goal will keep you hungry for more once you reach it. That's especially true in running. Accomplishing one running goal should be satisfying, yet also leave you eager to find out what else you're capable of. All of the work you did to meet the first goal will set you up for the next one.

Keeping a training log can help you meet your goals. You'll get great satisfaction and renewed motivation from seeing your progress in tangible form. You'll also be able to note patterns and have a record telling you what does and doesn't work for you.

You can keep a log with one of several apps or online platforms, or you can go old-school and maintain a handwritten log. Use whatever format you're most likely to update frequently (ideally, on each day that you run, while the details are fresh). Include whatever details are most meaningful to you, such as distance, pace, route, weather, how you felt, who you ran with, etc.

RUN WITH GOOD FORM: There's no one perfect running form. Watch the best runners in the world, and you'll see different arm carriages, degree of knee lift, number of steps taken per minute, etc. Everyone has a unique mix of strength, flexibility, bone structure, and other factors that affect how they run.

That said, if you look carefully at top runners, you'll see some important common elements among most of them. Good running form allows you to run the same pace with less effort, reduces your risk of injury, and simply makes running feel better. The basic elements of good running form include:

- 🐭 **Good alignment:** Have someone take photos or video of you running at your normal pace. Ideally, you'll be able to imagine a line connecting your head, shoulders, hips, and ankles. Running with these parts askew from one another makes you more inefficient and increases your risk of injury. A great mental cue to reset your alignment is to tell yourself to *run tall*. Thinking about that phrase should help you un-scrunch and straighten misaligned body parts.

- 🐭 **Setting a slight forward lean:** The goal here is a slight forward lean from your ankles. Bending forward from the waist is one of the most common form flaws new runners exhibit, and one of the most consequential. It puts an unnecessary strain on your lower back, hip flexors (muscles along the front of your legs), and shoulders—and keeps you from using the full power of your hamstrings and glutes. Not good!

- 🐭 **Landing under your center of mass:** Many beginners think the key to running better is

taking long strides. That approach often results in landing ahead of the center of your mass. As a result, you wind up running slower, because you're slightly braking the stride with each step. You're also absorbing more impact forces than is necessary. If you can see your heel strike the ground, you're probably overstriding.

- 🐭 **Relaxation:** This last trait of good form is harder to quantify than the others, but it's as important. Unnecessary tension in your face, neck, shoulders, hands, or anywhere else does nothing but sap your precious energy. Do a head-to-toe body scan occasionally to see if you're feeling tight anywhere. Shoulders and arms are most often the culprits here; drop your shoulders and loosely cup your hands to let go of the tension. And this may sound silly, but if your face feels strained and tense, smile. Doing so will reset things.

The good news is that you can improve in any of these areas in which you feel you might not be reaching your maximum potential. In chapter 5, we'll look at some basic exercises that will build your running-specific strength and flexibility.

There's also no one universally desirable cadence (also known as stride rate—the number of steps you take per minute when running). Ignore anyone who says all runners should have a cadence of 180.

There is, however, a cadence that's too low for most of us. When your stride rate is less than optimal, your form will suffer. You'll probably be overstriding, and contending with increased impact forces. You'll also probably not be running as fast as you could even if you're expending the same effort, because your feet are spending extra time on the ground rather than propelling you forward.

Most runners will run more efficiently and feel better doing so if they get their cadence above 160 steps per minute. (That is, 80 steps with each foot.) If you're below that number, experiment by trying for brief periods to set a cadence that's over 160. The best way to get a quicker cadence to stick is to hold it for a minute or two at a time on several consecutive runs. Get a sense of what that lighter, quicker turnover feels like. Eventually, a different movement pattern will be imprinted in your brain, and you can naturally start to extend the time that you hold it. This is a better approach than increasing your cadence for an entire run only once a week.

THINK LIKE AN EXPERIENCED RUNNER: You'll know you've "become" a runner when someone asks, "But what do you think about during all these miles?"

Beginning and experienced runners think differently. Or, more accurately, while all runners tend to have similar thoughts and sensations, experienced runners have learned how to use those thoughts and sensations to their benefit. So, here's some advice on shortening your learning curve. One survey found beginning runners focus on bodily sensations and reactions, especially their breathing, while running. Runners are often told "listen to your body," though paying too much attention to how you feel isn't helpful. You'll get overwhelmed by thoughts like "this is too hard" and "I can't do this."

Experienced runners, however, treat these signals as their body giving them information that can be acted upon. Rather than viewing heavy breathing as a sign of distress, they realize it most often means they've started too fast and need to slow a little. Similarly, instead of feeling fatigued and saying, "I'm really tired and only halfway done," experienced runners will say (or think), "Can I relax my shoulders and get rid of some tension?" "Am I running with good form?" "Why do I feel tired?" And, "What can I do about it?"

Another thing that experienced runners are good at is motivational self-talk—words or phrases you say to yourself to improve your confidence and focus. Motivational self-talk has been shown

to help one maintain a given pace and make one feel more relaxed. So, instead of thinking (or stating), "I can't keep this up," tell yourself, "Keep going," "You're doing great," "You can do this," etc. There's evidence that addressing yourself in the second person ("you") rather than first person ("I") improves performance, perhaps because it's distancing yourself from the situation.

Another mental strategy to learn is called "chunking," or mentally breaking a run into smaller segments. Instead of thinking *I've only done one mile and am already tired, and I have two more miles to go*, think, *Great, you're one-third done. Pretty soon you'll be through mile two, and then all you have to do is run one more mile.*

While you're learning these strategies, it's also a good idea to learn how to distract yourself, by attempting to expunge—or tamp down—unpleasant thoughts and sensations. Run with a chatty friend, think about your day, take in your surroundings, listen to music or podcasts, and so on. Find ways to make the run enjoyable and draw attention away from your breathing and tired muscles. Have confidence that, if you stick with it, running itself will soon become a source of pleasure.

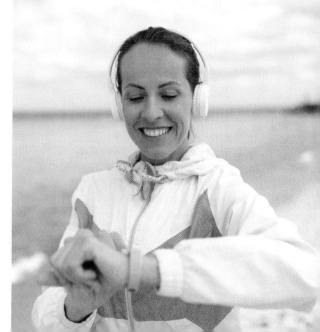

OVERCOMING COMMON NEW-RUNNER CHALLENGES

Although every runner is unique, many people face similar challenges when they first embark on making running a part of their routine. The following are some ways to overcome the most common roadblocks new runners encounter. Whichever of these issues and concerns you face, remember that millions of people have had to battle through the same things, yet are now regular runners. If they can do it, so can you!

CHALLENGE: I can't find the time.

SOLUTION: Lack of time is the top reason people give for not sticking to their running plans. That's understandable. We all seem so busy all the time.

The key to finding the time to run is to make it. That might sound facetious, but it really is the solution. Plan and schedule your runs like you do the other important things in your life. All you need is one segment of time two, three, or however many days a week you want to run. One of running's appeals is that you don't usually need much time for a good workout. You can get a lot accomplished with a few thirty-minute runs per week.

That magical block of running time might not present itself precisely at the exact time every day. That said, most surveys find that those who exercise in the morning more often stick with their plans. If you have a typical work schedule, there will probably be more claims on your time at 5:00 p.m. than at 5:00 a.m. Getting up a little earlier might not even cut into your sleep. If you know you have a run scheduled in the morning, you're more likely to use your time the night before wisely and get to bed at a more reasonable hour.

You have plenty of claims on your valuable time. When initially starting—and devoting a portion of time to running—you might need to be what may feel selfish, at least until you

establish the routine you want. But think of running as your "me" time! You do so much for others, and you deserve this time for yourself.

The thing is, eventually, you and others will realize your "me" time is really "for us" time. Running will make you healthier and happier, and you'll have that much more to give to others as a result.

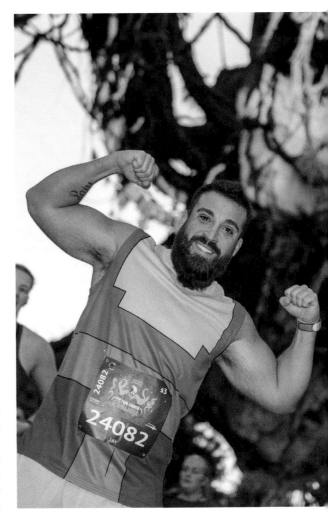

CHALLENGE: I'm inconsistent. I run for a few weeks, then miss a few weeks . . . and then run again and feel like I'm starting from scratch.

SOLUTION: We'll see in the next chapter that consistency is the key to enjoying and progressing in your running. So, how can you accomplish that?

First, evaluate your goals. (Or even more important, come up with some!) Do they meet the criteria described earlier in this chapter? If you struggle with consistency, the biggest reason could be because your goals aren't personally meaningful. You might feel like running is something that's just another obligation, not something you want to do. When you find a reason to run that really speaks to you, the day-to-day motivation gets a lot easier.

Second, find people to run with. Training partners are the greatest invention in running history. You'll develop amazing friendships through shared miles. And as in all good friendships, you'll know you can count on each other. It will be a lot easier to get out of bed, or show up after work, when you know a friend will be there waiting for you.

You might still have difficult days. All runners occasionally imagine themselves in the middle of a run, thinking *not today*. Try to "trick" yourself into running. Some common techniques to help you accomplish this are these:

🐭 **Change into your running clothes.** Tell yourself you're just going to do a little stretching. As your muscles start to warm and your mind gets clearer, you can start to picture yourself in motion and enjoying it.

🐭 **Go for a walk.** Tell yourself you don't have to run if you don't want to. Just get out the door and start moving. You'll usually feel like running soon enough. If not, no worries, enjoy your walk. That's not failing!

🐭 **Imagine yourself at the end of the day.** Do you want to head to bed happy with yourself? Or do you want to think about not doing what you intended? View your run as a part of the day you have control over. Think how much more satisfied you'll be if you get in just a short run.

CHALLENGE: I don't enjoy it.

SOLUTION: First, give yourself time to get fit. Wait until you can comfortably run for half an hour before deciding running's not your thing. Having that baseline running fitness will allow you to think about something besides being uncomfortable.

If you can comfortably run for half an hour but still don't enjoy it, look for ways to add pleasure to the routine. Can you listen to music or podcasts? Run more often in pleasant surroundings? Run with friends, a family member, your dog? Add variety (different paces or distances on different days instead of always doing the same run)?

Even the most die-hard runners don't find every run a peak lifetime experience. On difficult days, think about enjoyment in terms of satisfaction ("I did what I planned to do and am glad I stuck with it") more than momentary pleasure.

CHALLENGE: I get a lot of side stitches.

SOLUTION: Keep running!

Beginning runners seem to most often be affected by side stitches, which are sharp, stabbing pains below the ribs. It's believed that side stitches happen because your respiratory muscles get overwhelmed and go into spasm or cramp. That can happen because of heavy breathing and/or lack of running-specific midsection strength. But as you become a more experienced runner, your breathing will become more appropriately rhythmic, and you'll get better at maintaining a relaxed, efficient trunk position.

If you do get a side stitch, slow your pace however much is needed to get your breathing under control. Try to take some deep breaths in which you push your abdomen out while inhaling, rather than drawing your belly in while inhaling. Gently push on the painful area while you do this breathing centered on the belly.

CHALLENGE: It's too cold/hot/rainy/snowy/icy/windy to run.

SOLUTION: Some people will tell you, "There's no such thing as bad weather, just bad gear." That's taking things a little far. If you've ever run when it's ninety-five and humid, or minus twenty and windy, you know there is such a thing as bad weather.

The no-bad-weather quip is more applicable on less extreme days. However, the right high-quality running apparel will help you stay cooler when it's warm outside, and, conversely, warmer when it's cold . . . and drier when it's wet. In chapter 3 we'll look at how to select the right running gear for where you live.

But perhaps more important than gear when it comes to dealing with weather is your mindset. As you gain more experience as a runner, you'll better sense the weather is almost never as bad as it looks when you first gaze out the window. True, you might not always enjoy a given's day weather. But there's something satisfying about being the sort of person who doesn't let less-than-ideal conditions deter you (and knows that your lungs won't freeze in the cold).

Certainly, there are days where caution is warranted. Ice, lightning, extreme heat, and poor air quality can be dangerous. Those days are rare for most of us. And remember, there's always the treadmill.

CHALLENGE: I don't look like a runner.

SOLUTION: Do you run? Then you look like a runner.

Runners come in all shapes, sizes, colors, and ages. The days of the average runner being a skinny twenty-eight-year-old man are long past. Women make up more than half the field at most road races, and every age group is represented. Go watch a race, or just take note of all the people you see running over the next week, and you'll find all body types represented.

This isn't to downplay any self-consciousness you might have. Society's messages about body images can be paralyzing. But that's not what running is about. Running is full of welcoming people who are happy to have new members join the group. The few runners who look down at others for not being "real runners" are the outcasts, not you.

Wear whatever clothes you're comfortable in. If people judge negatively your appearance, that's their problem, not yours.

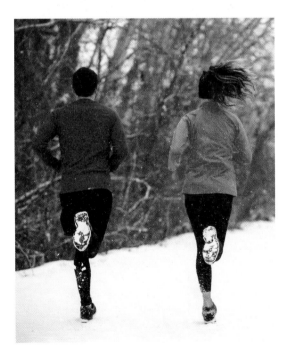

CHAPTER 2:
HOW TO BUILD ENDURANCE AND SPEED

If you've gone from being sedentary to being a regular runner, congratulations! You've taken the biggest step of all—joining the worldwide group of runners. The difference between you and those who win marathons is now much smaller than the difference between you and those who are inactive.

If you want to maintain your running routine, yet don't feel the need to go any farther and faster, that's completely fine. You're as much of a runner as people who run three times as far and are twice as fast. If you're happy with your running, that's all that matters.

Still, once they've taken that hardest, most important step of establishing the habit, many runners want to keep exploring. Runners tend to be can-do, goal-driven people. It's natural that some of them will want to see what happens if they start running more, or faster . . . or both. That curiosity often goes hand in hand with their desire to add the excitement of races to their running life.

Going farther and faster is what this chapter is about. We'll look at how to safely increase endurance and speed while keeping running fun and healthy.

CONSISTENCY IS KEY

The great Grete Waitz, who won more New York City Marathon titles (nine) than anyone else ever will, offered this advice to her fellow runners: hurry slowly.

The marriage of those two words perfectly captures how to succeed long-term as a runner. Hurry, in that you want to have a certain eagerness about your running; slowly, in that it's the gradual accumulation of proper efforts that builds fitness, week to week, month to month, season to season, year to year, even decade to decade. A low simmer of commitment and patience is something you can sustain physically, mentally, and logistically for the rest of your life.

The point of training isn't to get as tired as possible. (That's a good approach if your goal is to get hurt or burned-out.) The point is to apply a stimulus that will, temporarily, break your body down a little. Then, if you allow your body the proper recovery time, it will rebuild itself to be a little better at handling a similar stimulus. As Waitz noted, this is a slow process. No one run leads to sudden dramatic improvements. Think instead of someone dedicated to saving for retirement, with small but regular deposits that build on each other to create something substantial.

That's another way of saying the most successful runners are the most consistent runners. That's true whether your definition of success is improving your cardiovascular health, running a few races a year, staying at a good weight, setting personal bests for longest distance covered, adding years to your life (and life to your years), bolstering your mental health, expanding your social network, or all of the above. Consistency will always top getting all fired up for a short while, and then getting burned-out, and then getting fired up again, and then burned-out, and so on.

Consistency will also improve your endurance and speed without your doing anything other than being consistent. Simply maintaining a regular running schedule for most weeks of the year will probably improve your average running pace. Similarly, you'll find that what used to be a challenging distance to reach will become more like your everyday run. That's a sign that your endurance has improved.

When you feel your fitness improving, it's natural to think about what else you can do to gain endurance and speed. Let's look at how to take those next steps.

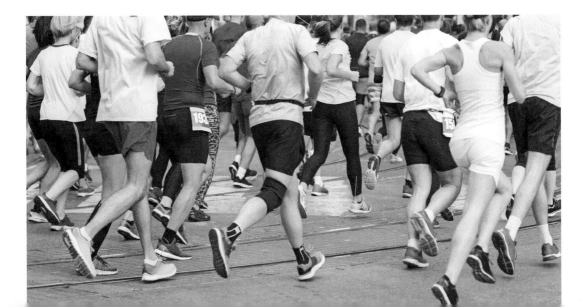

HOW TO USE THE RUNDISNEY TRAINING SCHEDULES

 Those who have a plan tend to do better than those who don't. My runDisney schedules offer you day-by-day training for every runDisney distance—whether you're just getting off the couch or are a competitive runner. You can add your success to the hundreds of thousands who have crossed the finish line using these programs.

As you look at the schedule each day, and check off each completed workout, you become accountable. You activate the cognitive brain each time you do this, which overrides the emotional subconscious brain that sends you negative hormones under stress.

The long workout is the key to the program. You'll start at a short distance and gradually increase, every other week, to race distance or an even slightly longer stretch. On the non-long-run weekends, only a short run is required—giving you more time for family and social activities.

Between long-weekend runs, the minimum workout is only thirty minutes every other day for most (and a bit more for time-goal runners).

My run-walk-run method can be adjusted to avoid three conditions I worry about runners confronting: pain, exhaustion, and puking. If you're stressed by any of these, take a reset walk for three minutes; then shorten the run segment and increase the frequency segment of the walk.

If you're having a bad day, just walk the distance of the long runs. You'll attain the same endurance level based upon the distance covered.

The full training programs are available at rundisney .com/running-training -programs/.

—Jeff Galloway,
Olympian and official
runDisney training consultant

HOW TO SAFELY INCREASE YOUR MILEAGE

Would you like to double your weekly mileage? Simple—go twice as far as you usually do however many days a week you run. At the end of the week, you'll have doubled your mileage.

Of course, at the end of the week you'll probably also be exhausted, sore, sick, sick of running, and maybe even injured. A crash training program of suddenly doubling your mileage ignores a key phrase from above: "If you allow your body the proper recovery time." Learning how to balance pushing your limits with the right amount of rest is the key to safely and enjoyably running more! Getting that balance right goes a long way toward avoiding injury. When you avoid injury, you can maintain the consistency that underlies true progress in running. (We'll look at avoiding injury in detail in chapter 5.)

So, how do you successfully start running more? You may have heard about the "10 percent rule," which says not to increase your mileage by more than 10 percent per week. For example, if you currently run twenty miles a week and want to do more, you would go no more than twenty-two miles the following week.

This "rule" has its merits . . . and it has caution baked into it, plus provides a precise directive on how much to safely increase your mileage. You could do worse than following it.

You could probably also do better: for starters, the figures "1 mile" and "10 percent" have no inherent meaning to your body. So, to call this advice a *rule* gives it more heft than it deserves.

It's also best not to consider it a *rule* because its implications vary greatly depending on your current mileage. If you're one of the tiny fraction of 1 percent of runners who cover a hundred miles a week, then yes, increasing by no more than 10 percent (in this case from 100 to 110 miles a week) makes good sense.

But what if you're a beginner who has successfully made it a habit to cover ten miles a week? You're enjoying your running, and you feel ready for more, so the next week you do . . . eleven miles.

The week after that it's 12.1 miles, followed by a 13.3-mile week. At that rate, it won't be until your eighth week that you finally get past twenty miles. For most people, this is like locking up your house every time you go next door for a few minutes—safe, but close to letting fear of something bad happening overwhelm everything else.

Here's a better way to safely increase your mileage: if you're running less than four times a week, add another day of running, with that day's run at the low end of your normal range. So, if you usually run fifteen miles a week in three days, add a day where you run approximately three miles. If you're running four or more days per week, try adding a mile or two to most of your runs.

Once you've made that jump, try two more tricks to make it stick. First, stay at that new level for a few weeks. Let your body adapt to this amount of running being the new normal. Then, after three weeks of increased mileage, take a "down" week—return to what had been your

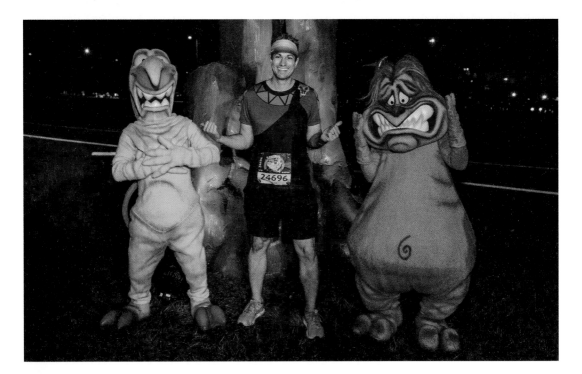

TOP 5 MISTAKES WHEN FOLLOWING THE OFFICIAL RUNDISNEY TRAINING SCHEDULES

 If you want to get the most out of my runDisney training schedules, avoid these common mistakes.

NOT DOING THE LONGER RUNS AT THE END OF THE TRAINING SCHEDULE. The last long run, about two weeks before the race, will set your endurance for race day—and help you avoid the fatigue wall. If you don't feel like running on that day, just walk the distance that is assigned. You'll build up the same endurance.

NOT DOING THE SHORT MAINTENANCE RUNS TWO DAYS EACH WEEK BETWEEN WEEKEND RUNS. The short runs sustain your running adaptations. If you don't do these, the long runs will become more and more difficult.

CHOOSING A MORE AGGRESSIVE SCHEDULE OR TIME GOAL THAN YOU'RE READY TO RUN. Use my "magic mile" prediction noted in the instructions of the training schedules provided to find a realistic goal—and do the training to prepare for that goal (see page 85).

TRAINING WITH A FAST FRIEND WHO INHERITED BETTER RUNNING GENETICS THAN YOU. Monitor your breathing when running with others. If you can't carry on a continuous conversation, walk to get your breathing under control and start running again with a more conservative strategy.

TRAINING TOO HARD DURING THE LAST WEEK BEFORE THE RACE. You only need to walk or gently run-walk-run (RWR) during the seven days leading up to the race. Hard training during this taper period won't improve your time but will increase your risk of injury.

—Jeff Galloway, Olympian and official runDisney training consultant

previous norm. This lighter week will give your body a chance to rest up and absorb the harder work you've been doing the past few weeks. After that down week, either return to your new normal, or take the same approach as before to make another jump in mileage.

It's normal to feel more tired when you increase your mileage. Your legs might feel "heavier" and it might take longer to feel lively when you run. When you're not running, you might feel a little lethargic and you might have an increased appetite that seems out of whack to the slight jump in mileage. These feelings will pass if you haven't bumped things up too much. However, if you get new, acute running-related pains, catch a cold that's otherwise inexplicable, or are running much, much slower than usual, those are signs that you've been overdoing it. Cut back to your previous mileage until these symptoms pass. Then try a new higher weekly mileage that's lower than your first attempts.

Adding more mileage in this patient, methodical but slightly ambitious way will almost always increase your endurance. Plus, you can get an additional boost by emphasizing a long run two or three times a month.

LONG LIVE THE LONG RUN

The weekend long run is a staple in millions of runners' lives. It's the cornerstone of the official runDisney training programs and most other programs for race distances of 10K and longer. Even people with no plans to race do a regular long run.

Having one run every week or two that's significantly longer provides a special oomph to your fitness that's hard to achieve otherwise. Once you get used to going long, you've become a more resilient runner. Your muscles are better able to fuel your running, your bones and soft tissues can maintain good form longer, your efficiency improves, you don't get sore as easily, and you can just overall hold up to challenging distances and paces much better. There are also psychological benefits to regularly going long: you gain experience in persevering, and your regular everyday runs don't seem nearly as challenging as they once did.

What constitutes a long run varies greatly, depending on your experience, goals, and current weekly mileage. To enjoyably complete a half marathon or marathon, you'll need to get used to long runs that are close to those race distances. In contrast, for someone running fifteen miles a week and focusing on 5Ks, a six-mile run is long enough to provide the needed endurance boost. In general, think of a long run as a run that's 20 to 50 percent longer than most of the other runs you do.

It's fine to do your long runs at your normal run pace, one where you can talk in full sentences. The challenge of the long run is covering the additional distance; you don't need to add the additional stress of trying to go faster than usual.

Although a weekend morning is when most people do their long runs, there's no law against going long Tuesdays at noon or Thursdays at dusk. Do your long runs when it works best and fits in with the rest of your life. Of course, for many

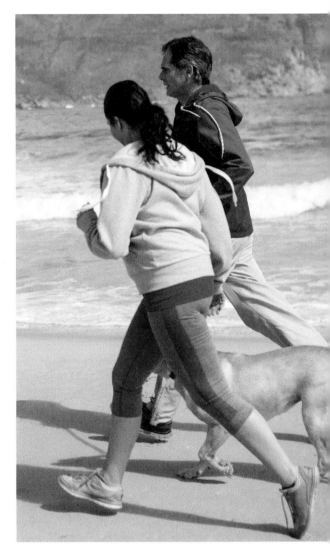

people, that will be a weekend morning. You're also more likely to find people to do your long runs with—one of the greatest pleasures in running, by the way—on weekends.

Consistent running—especially when you plug in regular long runs—almost always leads to getting faster. And once you've established that base, you can get even faster by occasionally upping your pace. Next, we'll look at the key types of runs that build your speed.

SPECIAL WORKOUTS TO BUILD YOUR SPEED

There are endless ways to do what's called speed work, purposely going faster than usual for at least part of a day's run. All of them help make running faster feel more natural—and all will help lower your times at all race distances.

But within all of these workouts, there are a few key types of faster running techniques that appear again and again. Each of these is done at a fairly precise effort that corresponds to the runner's race pace. While the benefits overlap among all speed workouts, each one covered is particularly effective when it comes to attaining a faster pace on race day.

You're under no obligation to ever do any of these workouts. You can run with great satisfaction and enjoyment the rest of your life solely with steady distance runs. But if you find yourself seeking to up your speed, these workouts will get you there. Race results aside, many runners find that doing these workouts adds an enjoyable challenge to their routine.

You can do these workouts wherever you find the best conditions for you. The track is still the go-to locale for many, because of the setup and predictability it offers. But GPS watches have made it a lot easier to take to roads or bike paths. These options are often more convenient, which means you're more likely to regularly do the workouts. (The same is true of treadmills.) Doing your faster workouts off the track also better prepares you for road races, with their turns, hills, and harder-than-a-track asphalt.

For all but the first type listed below (striders), you'll want to first begin a workout with a warm-up jog of one to three miles. Doing so will prime your cardiovascular system and, as the name implies, warm your muscles for the harder work ahead. After the workout, jog a mile or two. This post-workout cooldown helps your body return to normal better than just stopping right after a hard run. You'll feel better on subsequent runs if you do cooldowns.

STRIDERS: In running lingo, striders (or strides) are short accelerations done after a regular run, or as part of a warm-up before a hard workout or race. They're the perfect way to introduce planned, faster running workouts into your program. Striders improve your functional range of motion, foot speed, efficiency, muscular strength, and form. That's a huge payoff for something that's not taxing and that feels great during and after!

Striders are not sprints. Don't try to run them as fast as you can, and don't strain. Doing striders properly entails accelerating to about the pace you could hold for a mile, and then holding that effort for about a hundred meters (the length of a straightway on a track). Concentrate on staying relaxed and moving smoothly. After each strider, rest until you feel ready to run the next one with the right combination of quickness and ease.

A typical session is six to twelve striders after one of your daily runs. You can also incorporate them into the end of a normal run. With a mile or two to go, alternate twenty seconds fast with forty seconds of going easy several times. Start with one session each week, then feel free to do them as often as you'd like. Striders are invigorating, not exhausting, so you don't have to account for recovery time in the days after doing them. Striders are best done on a flat, level surface where you can concentrate on good form and quick feet.

SHORT PICK-UPS: Think of these as an extension of striders. Short pick-ups are done at about the same pace, but held for thirty to sixty seconds. They're more taxing than striders, but short enough to allow good running form at a fast pace and for your breathing to return to normal soon after each pick-up. Short pick-ups improve your running efficiency and provide good practice at staying relaxed at faster paces.

You can do short pick-ups as a conventional

workout, with a warm-up and cooldown. After warming up, run six to twelve pick-ups of between thirty and sixty seconds, with one minute of jogging in between. Or you can incorporate the pick-ups into the end of a normal run. If opting to do that, be sure to leave time for at least five minutes of jogging afterward.

TEMPO RUNS: A tempo run is done at the pace you could hold in a race for about an hour. A classic tempo workout begins with a one- or two-mile warm-up that's followed by a run of fifteen to thirty minutes at tempo pace, and then a cooldown. The pace should feel "comfortably hard"—you're working harder than usual, and concentrating more than you have to on a normal run. But you should still be able to speak in complete sentences if you had to.

Regular tempo runs are one of the best ways to run a faster half marathon or marathon once you have a good endurance base. They improve your ability to sustain a steady pace. They're also great practice at maintaining good running form as you tire. In addition, they provide great mental training—since you'll learn how to keep working hard as the urge to stop or slow mounts.

5K PACE REPEATS: You can accomplish a lot with just striders, short pick-ups, and tempo runs. But to get that little extra bit of improvement, especially for shorter road races like 5Ks and 10Ks, try workouts at a 5K-race pace. Doing repeated short runs at this effort level improves your heart's ability to pump a lot of blood, and improves the ability of your muscles to use the oxygen in that blood. As a result, you'll be able to sustain a faster pace when taking on the highly challenging 5K and 10K distances.

After warming up, do four to eight runs of two minutes to five minutes at your current 5K race pace. The total amount of hard work you should do is between two and three miles, or between half and all of your 5K time. For example, if you run a 5K in 30:00, you would aim to total between 15 and 30 minutes of running at a 5K-race pace by doing six three-minute repeats. Between those segments, and at a 5K race pace, do a recovery jog of two to three minutes each time.

Most runners find these workouts to be the most tiring. Your muscles, mind, and cardiovascular system will be working really hard. Don't do these workouts more than two or three times a month, and save them for the few months before a 5K or 10K you want to do really well in rather than doing them year-round. Give yourself a few days of easy running before and, especially, after. (There will be more on how to incorporate these and other fast workouts into a typical week coming up.)

HILL REPEATS: You've probably noticed that running fast uphill is hard. The extra work against gravity taxes your muscles and cardiovascular system, plus is mentally demanding. But that's why, if done correctly, hill repeats can build your speed, even though you might not be going that much faster than during a normal run on flat ground.

After warming up, do six to ten uphill repeats of a hill that takes you thirty to ninety seconds to climb at about 5K-race effort, not 5K-race pace. (If the best hill near you takes longer than that to transcend, just mark off a spot partway up it.) Jog down the hill for your recovery, taking care not to slam your feet into the ground! Runners more often get injured from the downhill jogs than the uphill spurts such workouts entail. The hill should be steep enough to be noticeably more challenging than flat ground, but not so steep that you can't run up it fast with good, erect form.

Longer hill repeats can be tougher to pull off. The jog down between repeats can last too long, cutting into the benefit of the workout. You also endure an awful lot of pounding on tired legs during those downhill jogs. If you're preparing for a race with long uphill segments, do your regular runs on similar courses, and work the uphill portions.

HOW TO CATCH UP WITH THE OFFICIAL RUNDISNEY TRAINING SCHEDULE

 Almost every runner misses a few workouts during the training season. By making a few adjustments, though, you can be ready to enjoy a race weekend and earn your medal!

If you miss one of the short maintenance runs, try to walk for fifteen to thirty minutes on that day and just continue with the schedule. While you should try to do all of the maintenance runs, if you miss one of the short ones say once every two weeks you'll still be okay.

If you miss a long run, be sure to do the maintenance runs on the schedule three days a week. On the day of the next scheduled long run, you can walk the first half or even the entire distance to catch up with the schedule. That's right—even walking the entire amount of the long run will give you all of the endurance based upon the distance that you complete. For example, if you miss the scheduled eleven-miler on week twelve of the beginner's half marathon schedule, be sure to do all of your thirty- to forty-five-minute runs until the 12.5-miler you set for week fourteen. It's a good idea to walk the first six miles of this workout. If you feel strong at that point, you can adjust your run-walk-run strategy to one that's easier to endure and finish the 12.5 miles.

To illustrate, if you've been using a thirty-second-run/thirty-second-walk strategy on long runs, do the last six miles at a run-fifteen-seconds/walk-thirty-seconds strategy, or another gentle configuration. But if you feel that any running would be too challenging at the halfway point, just walk the rest of the 12.5-mile workout. On the following long run (fourteen miles in this example), you should also use a gentle strategy for at least the first half.

—Jeff Galloway,
Olympian and official
runDisney training consultant

BUILDING A BASIC TRAINING SCHEDULE

Increasing your mileage, doing regular long runs, and adding speed workouts will make you faster and better able to cover long distances without severe fatigue. There can also be a psychological benefit to regularly doing different types of runs. Many runners find the variety refreshing. Knowing that your next four runs will be two "normal" runs plus a faster session and a long run can make you more eager to train than if all your runs are more or less the same.

It's crucial when adding any or all of these elements to keep the basic work/recovery premise in mind. You gain endurance and speed only if, after those most challenging runs, you allow your body time to absorb your hard work. That means following long runs and speed workouts with one or more recovery days. Cramming harder days together won't make you fitter or tougher—but

WHAT IF I DON'T MEET MY EXPECTATIONS?

When you're new to running, you can make big improvements really quickly. This is exciting! However, you also don't have a huge base of miles and running experience from which to judge your fitness, which can make setting appropriate goals difficult.

Conversely, if you've been running a long time, it can be harder to find ways to improve with the same leaps and bounds that you did when you started.

I think it's fair to be disappointed with your race results sometimes. There are lots of variables that can undercut your goals. Your body is an ever-changing organism, and as much as we'd like it to, it doesn't have mechanistic predictability. Basically, some days you just don't feel good! In addition, as you take on events and races that are of greater distance—such as a half marathon and a marathon—illness, injury, fueling, blisters, and stomach issues can all affect your results.

I like to keep some kind of record of my training in a logbook to notice patterns and analyze what does and doesn't work. You can customize what variables to track. For example, I like to note patterns in weekly mileage, sleep, recovery rate, split times, and hormone cycles. A journal is also a great place to map workout plans, hold race calendars, and keep track of long-term goals on a visual scale.

I personally find writing my goals down in hard copy to be a powerful driving force—and motivator.

After doing a race where you feel you haven't hit your target, pinpoint what went wrong. (Sometimes a vantage point other than your own helps here.) Decide how you can do it better, and acknowledge how much of it was or wasn't in your control. Talking to a training partner or coach is a good way to decide how to adjust the sails. They can tell you if they think you're skipping a step on the way to a goal, or decide if you need to switch race distances, change your timeline, or try a new workout approach. With reflection, awareness, creativity, and perspective, you should be able to tackle any race plan!

—*Molly Huddle,*
Olympian and American
record holder for 10,000
meters and the half marathon

will send your injury-risk chances soaring, leave your enthusiasm for running plummeting, and most likely put your payoff from workouts into the trash can. Even the best runners in the world follow their longest and hardest runs with days of easy running.

So how should you put these elements together? For starters, don't add more than one new variable at a time. If you're increasing your weekly mileage, make that your focus. If you're good with where your weekly mileage is and want to gain endurance, start increasing the length of one of those runs once a week. If you're set on weekly mileage and the distance of your long run, start adding faster workouts.

If you're new to speed workouts, start with one or two days of striders a week for two weeks. Then experiment with short pick-ups and tempo runs, but do no more than one of either once a week. For example, one week have a day of short pick-ups. Then the following week skip the short pick-ups, and do a tempo run. After at least a month of these more challenging workouts, you'll be ready to do 5K-race-pace repeats.

For all of the types of speed workouts covered, start at the lower end of the suggested workouts.

Once you've found which elements you want in a typical training week, look at your calendar to see where each makes the most sense. A typical week could include your longest run on the weekend and your hardest workout in the middle of the week. Between those days would be your normal, everyday runs.

Training programs shouldn't be written in stone. Weather, work, illness, unusual soreness or fatigue, and other factors affect when it's best to do your next long run or speed workout. With experience you'll learn to distinguish between when your body is really telling you it needs

another easy day and when your mind is just messing with you. When in doubt, start the warm-up portion of your workout. If by the end of it you feel no better than you did at the start, continue on at an easy pace and postpone the workout until your next planned run.

What constitutes a recovery day varies greatly and depends on the runner. It might mean a day of no exercise, possibly a run at an easy pace, or it might mean not running but doing some other form of exercise. As your endurance and speed increase, you can more often do short, easy runs on your recovery days. But you don't have to! One of the great things about running is experimenting to find your unique perfect balance of work and rest. You'll know you've hit your current sweet spot when you look forward to most of your runs at the same time your body's capabilities are improving.

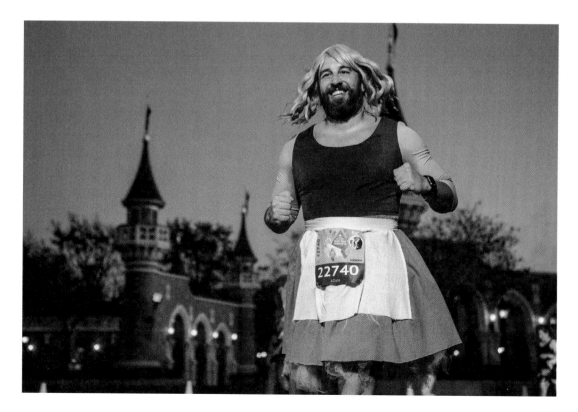

CHAPTER 3:
RUNNING SHOES AND OTHER GEAR

Running is rightfully known as a simple, accessible activity. You don't need to buy lots of equipment, learn how to use such equipment, or worry about your workout being ruined by broken equipment. You also don't need special surfaces or facilities. Get running shoes and apparel, and you're good to go pretty much anywhere in the world, at any time of the day.

That said, because running is so simple, it's really important that the few pieces of gear you need work well for you. The wrong shoes will make running feel like a chore, and could increase your risk of injury. Inferior clothing will make you hot when you want to be cool, or keep you cold when you want to be warm. Why battle blisters and chafing when you don't have to?

In this chapter, we'll cover the basic gear you need to enjoy your running, along with a few frills that can make your miles that much more rewarding (and in some cases, safer).

RUNNING SHOES: COMFORT IS KEY

Entire books have been written about running shoes. That's understandable, when you consider how central the right shoes are to enjoying your running. It's also understandable if you look at all the running shoe options out there and feel overwhelmed. Which of the hundreds of models of options out there should you choose?

As it turns out, finding the right shoes is pretty simple: go with the ones that mesh so well with your unique makeup that you practically don't notice them. We'll get to how to find those in a bit. But first, a little background on how not to choose running shoes.

Runners used to be told to select shoes largely on the basis of how much they pronate, which is another way of saying how much their feet roll in after landing when they run. The general model was that people who overpronate need stability features to control their excessive foot motion; people who land on the outside of their feet and stay on the outside while pushing off (this is known as supination) need highly flexible shoes. And those whose feet roll in a little should wear neutral shoes (middle-of-the-road models that are neither overly stiff nor super-flexible). Runners were told that the shape of their arch largely predicted where they were on the pronation spectrum, with flat-footed runners thought to need motion-control shoes and high-arched runners advised to lean toward the most flexible shoe models.

Most experts have now discarded this process. Sport-focused podiatrists point out that the shape of your arch when you're standing might not have anything to do with how your arch functions when you run. Research has found no relationship between degree of pronation, shoe type, and injury rate. One study, published in the *British Journal of Sports Medicine* in 2013, tracked almost one thousand beginning runners, with three equal subgroups of those classified as having pronated, supinated, or neutral feet. During the year of the study, the groups tracked had the same injury rate, even though all wore a neutral running shoe.

In other words, the runners who "should" have been in a more supportive or more flexible shoe got injured at the same rate the runners who were "supposed" to be in a neutral shoe did. In another study, women runners were randomly assigned to wear motion-control or neutral shoes while following a thirteen-week half marathon training program. Here, too, there were no differences in injury rates among the groups, even though most of the runners were in different types of shoes than what was recommended up to that point by the pronation-model-of-shoe-selection template.

So, if you go to a running store and the staff helps you select shoes on the basis of your arch shape and amount of pronation, *run* to another store!

How, then, do you know if a particular running shoe will work for you? It should feel like an extension of your feet. This is, admittedly, a more subjective standard than how high your arches are or how much you pronate, but it's backed by research. When runners select shoes on the basis of what feels best, they don't get injured as often.

Runners describe this sort of comfort by saying things like, "The shoes got out of my way" or "I realized I wasn't thinking about the shoes." Those sorts of descriptions indicate that the shoe is working in sync with the runner's form, rather than causing changes to the runner's gait. For many runners, it's a Goldilocks sensation—something that's not too light or too heavy, not too restrictive or too flexible, not too high or too low, and not too cushioned or too firm.

You can see that this more subjective (but better) way of finding shoes depends on how several aspects of the shoe work together. That's why it's imperative to try on several models, from several brands, to find the shoes that will work best for you. A good running store will encourage you to spend as much time as you need to start winnowing your choices. If there's not a good running store near you, order several models from an online retailer that allows free returns.

Here's an important point: the comfort factor should be ascertained when you're running, not walking in a selected shoe. As their name implies, running shoes are made for running. They might feel great when you step into them and take a few steps, but that tells you almost nothing about how they'll work for you once you're doing what they're made for. After all, you wouldn't select a cycling or mountaineering shoe on the basis of how comfortable it is when you walk around the store. Do short test runs in any shoes that pass the initial feels-good-to-have-on test.

The more you run, the more you'll develop this intuitive sense of whether a given running shoe will work for you. Beginning runners who are unsure can default to neutral shoes until they learn more about themselves out on the course.

A FEW OTHER SHOE-BUYING TIPS

- Allow about a thumb's-width space between the end of the shoe and the end of your longest toe (which might be your second toe). For many people, accounting for that little bit of room will mean going up half a size from their street shoes.
- Bring a few pairs of your running socks with you when you try on shoes. You might find that some shoes are too tight in thicker socks, or too loose in thinner socks.
- If possible, try on shoes later in the day, by which time your feet may have expanded a little bit. This step will help make sure the fit will accommodate your feet swelling during longer runs.

RUNNING SHOE BASICS

It's good to know a little about running shoe construction. Having an idea about what works for you in terms of weight, height, and other elements allows you to quickly determine whether a given shoe is worth investigating. Here are the key parts of a shoe that, together, make one running shoe different from another.

UPPER: This is the part of the shoe that covers the top of your foot. High-quality shoes will have an upper part that neither irritates nor constrains your foot. Many uppers are now seamless or at least constructed with flexible material that won't create abrasions. At the same time, you want to make sure that when you try on shoes, the upper is adaptable to your preferred lacing pattern. Uppers that are "sloppy"—that make it hard to feel like your foot is comfortably held in place over the shoe—will result in excess motion with every stride.

MIDSOLE: This is the material between the upper and bottom of the shoe that provides cushioning. Midsoles can range from very soft to very firm, and from very high to almost nonexistent (more on that part in a moment). Most shoe companies use a proprietary material for their midsoles, and will tweak the height and firmness of the material depending on the shoe. That's why it's so important to try on a variety of shoe brands to find the ones that feel best suited to your unique needs.

Remember that what feels like a comfortable amount of cushioning when you first step into a shoe can become cumbersome after a few miles of running.

OUTSOLE: This is the bottom part of the shoe that hits the ground. Most outsoles are made of some form of rubber, with what's known as blown rubber being used when reducing the weight of the shoe is a priority. The trade-off for that weight saving is that blown rubber tends to wear out more quickly than heavier carbon rubber.

Two important things here: Make sure the pattern of the outsole is appropriate for your running gait and the surfaces you do most of your running on. To reduce weight, some shoes have rubber over only part of the midsole. If your feet strike the ground other than where the outsole is strongest, you'll sacrifice traction and will land directly on the midsole, which will make the shoe's cushioning deteriorate quicker.

Outsoles on shoes designed primarily for road running usually have small lugs to help with traction, although they can also be almost smooth. Trail running shoes usually have more cleat-like outsoles to help propel you through dirt, grass, mud, etc. The latter don't feel all that great when you wear them on hard surfaces.

LAST: This is the shape of the material that attaches the upper to the midsole. Lasts can be straight, semi-curved, or curved, depending on what the shoe is designed for. Generally speaking, shoes made for faster running have a more curved last. Finding a last that will allow your foot to move as it wants to is a key element in choosing the right running shoe.

STACK HEIGHT: This pertains to how far above the ground your foot is when it's inside the shoe. Stack height is primarily a function of how tall the midsole is, but the thickness of the outsole and the interior construction of the shoe also play a part.

As with the amount of cushioning and stability in a shoe, what stack height feels best varies greatly from runner to runner. Some runners like a relatively low stack height because they like to better "feel" the ground. Others prefer a plush, relatively high stack height for the sensation of running on clouds that it provides. You definitely need to run rather than stand or walk in a pair of running shoes to determine if its stack height will feel natural to you.

HEEL-TO-TOE DROP: The difference in stack height between the back and front of the shoe is measured by this. Most mainstream running shoes have a heel-to-toe drop between four and twelve millimeters.

Proponents of a slight (or nonexistent) heel-to-toe drop say that more level shoes encourage a more natural running form. After all, when you run barefoot, the heel-to-top drop is zero. Others say that a moderate heel-to-toe drop accounts for the fact that most people first strike the ground with their heels, and a slanted construction better allows your foot to roll through the gait cycle.

Shoes with a smaller heel-to-toe drop tend to work your calves and Achilles tendons harder than more slanted shoes. Wearing shoes with a higher drop can result in higher impact forces on your knees. Keep these basic parameters in mind if you have a history of injury to either area. As with the other elements of a shoe, testing a variety of heel-to-toe drops will give you an idea of which fit feels most natural to you.

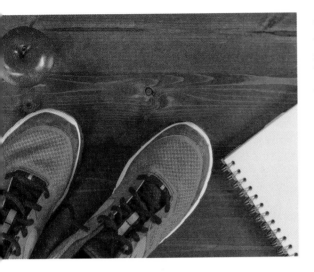

WEIGHT: All of these aspects, plus the materials the shoe's made of, determine its weight. For most runners, there's a sweet spot between the shoe being light enough so that it doesn't feel clunky and still being substantial enough so that it doesn't feel like you're running in bedroom slippers.

One of the great features of modern running shoes is that they're able to offer lots of comfortable cushioning without being as heavy as they were even a decade ago. So, consider yourself fortunate that you can probably find a shoe with a midsole, outsole, stack height, etc. that works for you at a weight that won't make running too laborious.

A FEW OTHER POINTS ABOUT SHOES

Many runners rotate among two or more pairs of shoes at a time. Doing so is a good idea for two reasons. First, wearing different shoes slightly changes how your body absorbs the impact stress of running. It's widely believed that most running injuries are caused by a body part not being able to withstand the repetitive stress it's subjected to. So, the thinking goes, by changing how that stress is distributed, you can lower the risk of any one body part crossing its threshold.

This line of thinking isn't just theoretical. In one twenty-two-week study, runners who rotated three running shoe models over this period had a 39 percent lower rate of injury than runners who always wore the same shoe.

The other reason to consider having more than one pair of shoes? Doing so might extend the life of your shoes. Just like you, shoes appreciate a little rest and recovery after long or hard efforts. Midsole compression is a big cause of running shoes going from feeling great to feeling like bricks. Also, uppers on shoes that are still wet from sweat or rain are more likely to tear. From this perspective, buying two or three pairs of running shoes might seem like a greater financial outlay, but it should eventually save you money (especially if it leads to less injury and rehab bills).

If you go this route, look for models that are similar to your main shoe, in terms of midsole firmness, last, stack height, etc. As always, you want the other shoes to feel like they disappear on your feet. There will still be enough subtle differences in how you run in different models to lessen your injury risk.

Most running shoes come with a removable insole. Some runners like to replace them with more cushioned insoles. Whether you should do this or not is a judgment call. Over-the-counter insoles are often more comfortable than the at times flimsy insoles that come with shoes. But that extra layer of cushioning could affect whether the shoe meets the Goldilocks standard of comfort touched on earlier. In addition, these insoles might not fit the inside of a given shoe as well as the insole that came with the shoe. Heavier runners and runners with chronic foot injuries most often appreciate these over-the-counter insoles. If that's you, don't be afraid to experiment. You'll usually want to use the cushier insole instead of adding it to the insole that came with the shoe; using both can make the shoe too tight.

Experiment with differing lacing patterns to find the one that keeps your shoes snug throughout a run without causing discomfort across the top of your foot. The tongues of most shoes have a tab that you can—but don't have to—run the laces through. Generally speaking, people with wider feet will want to leave their laces out of this tab, while runners with narrower feet can benefit from the extra closure across the top of their feet.

Lace-lock devices can help if your shoes regularly loosen or come untied over the course of a run. And don't be afraid to put in different laces than those that came with your shoes. An eternal mystery in the running community is why so many shoes come with laces that, even after double knotting, are still long enough to trip over. (Another solution is to tuck the ends of the laces under the laces by the base of your toes.)

If you live where snow and ice on the roads are a reality, consider getting traction devices for your shoes. Sure, you could run on a treadmill all winter. But most runners find that boring and want to be outside. As noted earlier, doing too much of your training on a treadmill can make "normal" running feel odd when heading back outdoors for something like running a half marathon through Magic Kingdom Park.

There are several running-specific versions of these devices that fit over the outsole of your shoes. They do a great job reducing slipping and sliding (and falling!) on slick wintry roads or other surfaces. The improved traction means not only that you have a safer, less frustrating run, but also that you won't be as sore or strained afterward.

When should you stop wearing a given pair of running shoes? You'll often hear shoes should last from three hundred to five hundred miles. But don't be bound by that dictum (which, by the way, has been stated for decades, even though shoes supposedly get better year after year after year). Some runners can get up to a thousand miles out of a pair of shoes, while others are particularly rough on their trainers and need a new pair every month or two. You'll know it's time to think about retiring shoes when you start noticing them more on your runs. That's an indication the cushioning has decreased significantly or that the shoe's structure has changed due to use.

Finally, it's important to keep running shoes in perspective. Although the right running shoes can reduce your injury risk, there's no evidence that running shoes will unilaterally prevent injury. If you repeatedly make some of the training errors that can lead to injury, it doesn't matter what's on your feet—you'll eventually get hurt! (We'll look at those errors and how to avoid them in chapter 5.) In addition, while the wrong running shoes might slow you down, the right running shoes can't do more than allow you to be as fast as you're capable of at any one time.

You wouldn't think the perfect swimsuit would magically make you an Olympic swimmer, or that a custom-fitted bike seat would make you a world-beating cyclist. Consider your running shoes tools for a job. Find the right tool, and your work as a runner will be a lot more enjoyable.

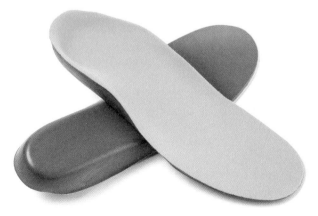

DRESSING FOR SUCCESS: RUNNING APPAREL BASICS

It's true that the right pair of shoes is the one absolute—the gear that's a necessity for enjoyable running. But good apparel will also go a long way to, well, helping you comfortably run a long way.

Modern running clothing is a marvel. It's lightweight but warm; it works well in a wide range of weather conditions; it gives in all the right places without getting in your way. And some of it even doesn't stink after several runs!

Most of the good stuff will be made of what are known as microfibers—specially made polyester and other fabrics that wick moisture to their surface. When it's hot and that moisture is sweat, you'll stay cooler and not be as troubled by clingy clothing. When it's cold and that moisture is sweat, you'll stay warmer. Although most running gear isn't waterproof—that would make it too heavy—the exterior of good apparel will deflect a reasonable amount of rain or snow.

An alternative material is merino wool. It's non-itchy, a great insulator, has a superb warmth-to-weight ratio, and doesn't trap odors like unnatural fabrics tend to. Merino's biggest drawback is that, once its fibers are saturated with sweat, they stay wet for a long time. So, it's best for running in moderate to cold weather.

Dress for how warm you'll be ten to fifteen minutes into your run. That's pretty easy to do when the temperature is above, say, fifty-five or sixty degrees Fahrenheit, when there isn't that initial *Brrr* factor to overcome. On colder days, resist the urge to bundle up as if you'll be standing at a bus stop. Of course, you can always take a top layer off if you get too warm. But it's better to feel unencumbered and properly dressed for the bulk of your run. One great thing about today's running apparel is that they're perfect for layering. Their light-but-warm qualities often keep one warm enough within a few minutes on cold days, but not roasting or sweating heavily half an hour later.

Wear what you'll be most comfortable in! That's good guidance not only from a physical perspective, but from a psychological perspective as well. Just because other runners like to show a lot of skin, or favor gear that leaves little doubt about their body shape, you're not obligated to. High-quality running apparel is available across the board from the skintight to free-flowing.

The same thing goes for colors and styles. If hot pink is your thing, flaunt it. If you like understated athleisure wear, don it. Long shorts, short shorts, full-length pants, Capri tights, double duty pullovers, muscle tops—you can find good gear in whatever look you like best. There's nothing wrong with wanting to look good when you run.

Here's quick guidance on the main types of apparel.

TOPS: If you live where there are four full seasons, you'll want at least one sleeveless top, a short-sleeve shirt, a long-sleeve shirt, and a warmer outer layer, such as a quarter-zip top, a pullover, or a jacket. That arsenal allows several permutations—short sleeves over a base layer in brisk-but-not-freezing weather, a light long-sleeve top under an outer layer on colder days, etc.

BOTTOMS: Again, wear whatever style you want. Every imaginable length and close-fittedness of short is available in good material. Most runners prefer having a few pairs of varying lengths: longer pairs for cooler weather and trail runs, and shorter ones for hot days and races.

Try to find shorts you like with one or more secure pockets. Who doesn't like pockets? They're good for keys, phones, credit cards, money, food, and more. The flimsy internal pockets of old, out of which many a car key disappeared and was forever lost, have been replaced by unobtrusive side or back-zippered pockets. (You can also still find internal pockets, but they now can be sealed much better.)

HOW TO CHOOSE A SPORTS BRA

Runners come in all body sizes. As noted in chapter 1, if you run, you're a runner. These days, it should be pretty easy to find a sports bra that provides the right support and comfort for your unique needs.

If you have high-support needs, look for underwires and individual cup molding. Thicker H-straps—rather than racer-back or thin-strap styles—are more supportive. You might also prefer a non-chafing hook or zip closure, so that you don't have to squeeze the bra on and then wrestle the sweaty version off post-run. Heading to your local running store to get direction on fit and what brands will likely best meet your needs is a good idea.

Many women with low-support needs favor a simple bra, often with a racer-back design and medium to high coverage. A bra like this is comfortable enough to run in without a shirt on hot days, if that's your preference.

In general, soft, moisture-wicking fabric is important. It's helpful if a bra has pockets for things like a nutrition gel or a phone. Some have a storage hack to stash larger items like a phone or gel in the bra top anyway, so items don't bounce around in there the way they do in a shirt or shorts pocket.

Larger apparel manufacturers make a variety of bras, but you can also find brands that focus on runners with special needs—such as those who need high support or run while pregnant.

—Molly Huddle,
Olympian and American
record holder for 10,000
meters and the half marathon

A good pair of running pants or tights will make winter running so much more enjoyable. Modern pants strike a nice balance between modesty and performance—they're looser from the knee up but tapered toward the ankle. If you live in a wet climate, consider paying a little extra for water-repellent materials.

If you live where there are a lot of in-between weather days, Capri tights or half tights are a great addition. As with shorts and pants/tights, try to find ones with functional pockets.

UNDERWEAR: Most running pants don't have a built-in liner, so you'll usually want to wear underwear or running shorts when you run in them. There are lots of good options for performance underwear. Cotton isn't king once it gets wet with sweat on a wintry day, and you find yourself turning into the wind. Look for micro-fiber underwear that won't restrict your gait and that has only a few seams (meaning fewer opportunities for chafing). Blends containing merino wool add extra warmth for the coldest runs of the year.

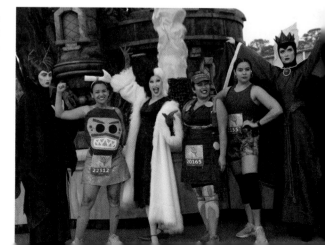

Whether to wear underwear when you run in shorts with a liner is a matter of personal preference. Try both options to see which is better for you. If you're a heavy sweater, you might find that you stay cooler going with just the liner of the shorts. On the other hand, if you have problems with chafing in the area on sweaty runs, underwear can help.

SOCKS: One aspect of socks is nonnegotiable; everything else is up to you. The nonnegotiable part is to avoid running in cotton socks. Most high-quality running socks are made of polyester microfibers. Unlike cotton, these fabrics wick moisture to the surface of the sock, resulting in greater comfort and less chance of blistering and infections such as athlete's foot. Merino wool socks are especially good at reducing friction and blisters, but can retain moisture if you sweat heavily. In colder conditions, a merino/microfiber blend adds welcome warmth.

Other than not wearing cotton, do what you want—short or long, thin or thick, boring or bold colors. It's good to have a variety of lengths and thicknesses. You might want your entire lower leg exposed in the summer, but covered in the winter. You might appreciate a calf-length sock if you're

running trails and don't want twigs and the like scraping your ankles. You might also find that different shoes in the same size fit best depending on the thickness of the sock.

HATS AND GLOVES: You probably already have a good hat for winter running. What you want is one that's close-fitting but not tundra-worthy heavy—and, of course, made to trap in warmth while moving moisture to the surface. Much of the heat you generate running is lost from your head, so while you want to keep your ears covered, you don't want something on top so heavy that you'll start sweating profusely.

Your fingers can get cold at what might seem like surprisingly moderate temperatures. It's not uncommon to see runners in shorts and a light long-sleeve top wearing gloves. Good-quality running gloves made of microfibers will keep your hands comfortable over a wide range of conditions, and are worth the investment. Some have tactile features on the thumbs and index fingers to help you manipulate your phone, watch, and other gadgets. If you regularly run in below-freezing temperatures, you'll probably want a pair of running mittens. On the harshest days, you can wear them over your running gloves.

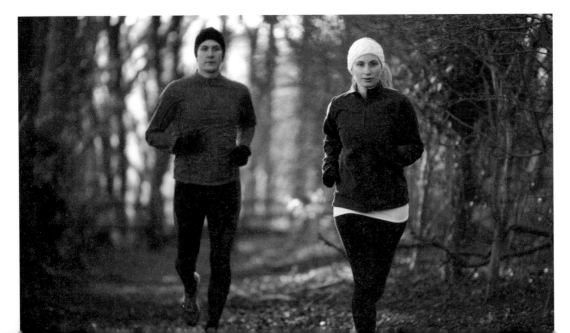

BEYOND THE BASICS

You've probably seen runners wearing knee-length compression socks or compression calf sleeves. Compression tights and tops are also popular, thanks to promises that they improve performance by returning more blood to your heart (which, theoretically, would then make more oxygen available for your body to draw from).

The jury is still out on those claims. So far, the best evidence indicates compression gear's effectiveness as a recovery tool after you run. Socks and tights with graduated pressure—reducing from the feet and ankles up the legs to the hips—have been shown to lessen post-run muscle soreness and perceived fatigue. If your muscles feel less fatigued, then you're able to return to normal running sooner after an especially long or hard run. Compression socks are also a good choice when you fly to races, because they can reduce stiffness and swelling around your ankles.

Sunglasses and caps are worth considering. They not only protect you from ultraviolet rays, but also can make you feel cooler on especially sunny days. (Because of solar radiation, the same temperature in the bright sun will feel warmer than on a cloudy day.) You don't have to break the bank to find a sturdy yet pliable pair of sunglasses that will protect your eyes and stay in place. For caps, many runners prefer trucker-style hats, because of the wide, long brims. Look for caps with mesh ventilation up top to allow heat to escape.

If you're among the millions of runners who like to listen to music, podcasts, or audiobooks while getting in their miles, you probably already have found earphones that work for you. So, the main point to make here is this: Keep the volume down! You should always be able to hear what's going on around you. It's not just a matter of safety (hearing vehicles, potential attackers, etc.) but also being courteous to runners, cyclists, and others who might give a heads-up that they're approaching from behind and assume you can hear them. Keeping the volume reasonable will also protect your hearing in the long run.

Two items that aren't gear but that go on your body merit mention: sunscreen and anti-chafing lubricants. We've all been advised to wear sunscreen when we'll be outside for more than a few minutes. But, as with driving and texting, many of us don't always do the right thing. Research shows that even people with good intentions usually don't apply enough sunscreen.

Dermatologists recommend using a sunscreen with a sun protection factor (SPF) of 30 to 50. Look for broad-spectrum products (meaning they block UVA and UVB rays) that have physical blockers like zinc oxide, which stay on your skin, rather than chemical blockers, which can be absorbed by your skin. Half an hour before your run, apply one ounce—the amount a shot glass would hold—over any area of skin that will be exposed during your run. Do so regardless of how cloudy or sunny it might be. There's no compelling evidence that lathering up will impede your sweating or otherwise cause you to be hotter than you otherwise would be.

There's no shame in chafing. Even very thin runners can generate enough friction to cause skin irritation, especially on hot days. If you chafe, apply one of the many sport-specific lubricants to your usual irksome areas. You might find that you're fine running without these products on shorter runs, but benefit from them on longer runs. When in doubt, use the lubricant. The last few miles of long runs can be challenging enough without the distracting discomfort of sweaty, raw skin.

We'll look at fuel belts and handheld bottles in the next chapter.

RUNNING SAFETY

 The main safety concerns for running outside are steering clear of vehicular and bike traffic, avoiding people or situations that could be dangerous, and finding help if you sustain a mid-run injury or encounter other kinds of medical issues.

I recommend carrying a phone in case you have an emergency. You can protect your phone in a runner-friendly waterproof holder.

Stay aware of your surroundings. If you listen to anything (music, podcasts, etc.) while running, keep only one earbud in so you can still hear things around you. It's a good idea to run facing traffic, and aim for routes with sidewalks or car-free trails rather than roadsides, if possible. A good tip when crossing driveways and intersections is to make eye contact with drivers before crossing in front of a vehicle at any point. A good rule is to assume no one sees you!

You may ideally want to avoid running in the dark and opt for a treadmill run instead, but it's necessary sometimes to get miles done at night or before sunrise. (This is better than no run at all!) On such runs, wear reflective clothes, or a reflective vest over your gear. You can also buy blinking-light features/reflectors that clip on to clothes as well as headlamps made for runners, which are also a great way to see and avoid potholes and curbs on dark roads.

As a woman running alone, I usually avoid isolated locales or areas I'm not familiar with. If possible, I do a well-lit loop or run with a friend. And to the dog owners out there, run with your pet if you're able to; they can be a loyal and protective buddy as well!

Another piece of gear that can address safety needs is a GPS watch with a cell signal. It allows you to leave your phone at home but still message via the watch if, for example, you're injured and would rather call for a ride than further aggravate something. It's also a good idea to have some form of identification on you when you head out the door. Running ID bracelets are a good way to carry this info without feeling overly burdened by gear. An alternative: I like to slip a credit card or ID into my phone case when I head out alone.

These are basic precautions, and aren't meant to worry you. The goal is for you to be aware, yet make sure safety concerns aren't preventing you from getting out the door and accomplishing your run!

—Molly Huddle,
Olympian and American
record holder for 10,000
meters and the half marathon

WATCH IT: ONE MORE KEY WEARABLE

A good running watch is your most important item other than shoes and clothing. If nothing else, you'll use it to track segments if you're using the run-walk-run method.

You can still find basic watches that have a stopwatch function, a lap timer, and a countdown timer, but no GPS or other high-tech features. These simple watches are more than adequate if you don't need or want to know precisely how fast and far you're going.

Of course, most runners find the additional data helpful. Seeing how far you've run, or how fast you're going, can be an added incentive. One of running's appeals is its objectivity—it's easy to track your improvements in endurance and speed. GPS watches make monitoring those metrics simple, both while you're running and over time when checking past performances. More advanced smart watches can also tell you things like your heart rate, your cadence (the number of steps you take per minute), and provide other feedback on your running form, such as your ground contact time with each foot strike (generally, shorter is better). Route stats such as total elevation gain can be useful as well if you're preparing for a hilly race, or if you just want a good explanation for why your last run was perhaps slower than usual.

What's worth tracking? Whatever you find helpful. Most runners like to know (and tell others!) their distance and pace. Tracking your heart rate can help you not overextend yourself, especially early in a run. Data on various aspects of your form can help you run efficiently, if you know what to do with what you see.

But as you probably know from other areas of your life, more data isn't necessarily better if you don't know what to make of it, or if it keeps you from focusing on fundamentals. Don't become a slave to running data, and don't spend your runs staring at your watch. Never work harder than your body is telling you it wants to just because your watch says you're going slower than some arbitrary figure, such as 10:00 per mile. Instead, use the data to help you progress toward your goals. Focus on general trends over time, not the inevitable day-to-day variations.

If you go the high-tech, run-data route, should you share your run on platforms such as Strava, the social fitness network, or post watch selfies on Instagram? That's a judgment call. If posting your runs will motivate you to be more consistent, go

for it. Be sure, however, that you don't run farther or faster than you should on any one day just to make a run look better on social media. Training is a means to an end—in this case, nailing your runDisney goal. Take pride in your training, but let your race results do the real talking.

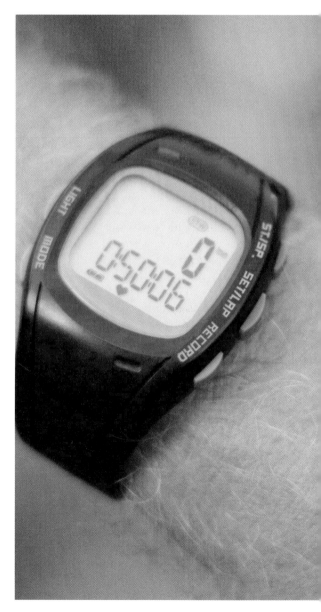

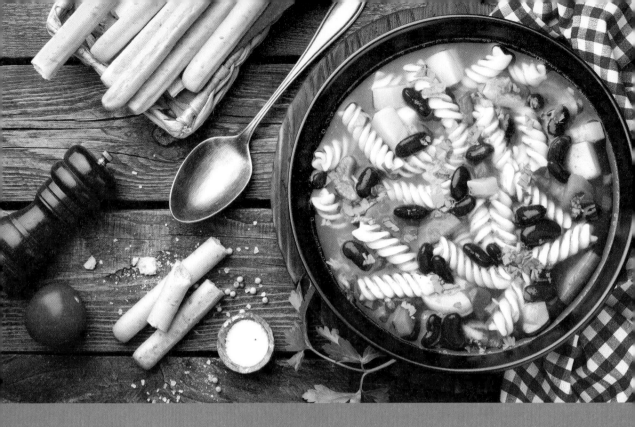

CHAPTER 4:
WHAT TO EAT AND DRINK

The quickest way to start an argument among runners is to talk about diet. Most runners will agree to disagree about training programs, shoes, even the meaning of life. But when it comes to what runners should eat and drink? Them's fightin' words!

Some of this cantankerousness stems from sincerity. One runner has found what works for her unique metabolism and innards, and wants to share this discovery with others. Most of the raised hackles, however, are based on a funda-mental misconception about the role nutrition plays in running. Encouraged by endless market-ing, we've been led to believe that we can eat our way to victory. Olympic runners are asked, "What do you eat?" much more often than "How do you train?"

As with workouts and gear, there's no "secret" or "magic" food, and no "diet hack" that's going to make you able to run dramatically farther and faster. Proper running nutrition consists of con-sistently good, unflashy choices that support your

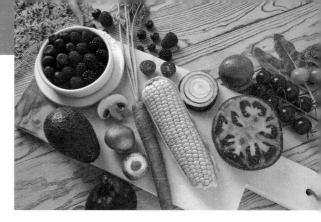

health and allow you to train as hard as you want. In this chapter, we'll look at what that means in terms of your daily dietary selections, as well as running-specific matters. We'll also see how to lose weight from running while still fueling your training.

A GOOD RUNNING DIET IS SIMPLY A GOOD DIET

In large part, what constitutes a good diet for runners is the same as what constitutes a good diet, period! You won't last long as a runner with an unhealthy diet, especially those of us who aren't as young as we used to be. Sure, you can "get away" with being a runner who doesn't think about your food, just like you can get away with running a half marathon without a sound training program. But neither will allow you to be your best.

You may have heard some version of the old runner's saying, "If the furnace is hot enough, it will burn anything." This is taken to mean that, if you run enough, you can eat whatever you want because it's all going to get burned away. That's true, more or less, in terms of weight gain. Few of us, however, run so much that we have to force ourselves to eat enough to keep weight on.

More important, the furnace metaphor ignores the quality of fuel. A good running diet provides the nutrients that allow your body to hold up to the demands of your training. These demands include:

🦶 Restocking your muscles' energy stores, via the intake of carbohydrates.

🦶 Repairing your muscles after hard or long runs, via protein and amino acids.

🦶 Maintaining a high red blood cell count, via iron and B vitamins.

🦶 Keeping your immune system strong, via vitamins.

🦶 Keeping your bones strong, via minerals.

🦶 Maintaining healthy hormonal levels, via good fats and enough calories.

Shortchanging these bodily needs means you won't be able to run as far and as fast as you're able. Or you'll often get sick, or get injured repeatedly . . . or possibly all of the above.

What does all of this mean in practical terms? Aim to meet the above big-picture needs daily. Doing so will mean having a well-rounded diet: a balance of nutrient-dense carbohydrates, lean proteins, and healthier fats (mostly not saturated fats); lots of fresh produce; a minimal amount of processed foods; and variety within the broad food categories (for example, several types of grain and seed foods rather than just pasta, and a range of produce colors that span the spectrum rather than just bananas and broccoli, etc.).

This approach to eating as a runner not only meets your nutritional needs, but is also a way of thinking about food in terms of choices rather than sacrifices. It gets you away from thinking of some foods as forbidden, or viewing food through a good/bad filter. It leaves room for indulgence, personal preferences, sensitivities, convenience, sometimes even getting together with others. For example, allowing yourself to

CAN YOU BE A NO-MEAT ATHLETE?

It's outside the scope of this book to look at why you might want to be a vegetarian or vegan. If you have made that choice, or are considering it, will you be able to run your best?

Yes, if you've done your homework. Well-planned vegetarian and vegan diets won't lead to protein deficiency. Research comparing meat-eating athletes to vegetarians has found no difference in thigh muscle size and lung function between the two groups.

Good iron levels are essential in running. Iron produces hemoglobin, a red blood cell component responsible for transmitting oxygen to your muscles. When your iron stores are low, a given pace will feel more difficult. You might also feel chronically fatigued, which undermines a lot of the pleasure of running and can seriously cut into your motivation.

Most people eating a typical American diet get adequate iron through meat and other animal sources of food. Iron absorption from plant sources is about half that from animal sources, so vegetarians and vegans need to put a little more care into meal planning. You'll want to regularly emphasize iron-rich plant options such as kale and spinach.

be "flexible" in social situations and occasionally having meals with others you might not make for yourself.

Try not to avoid entire food groups unless you have credible evidence that you should. To take one example, only 1 percent of people in North America and Europe have celiac disease, which makes their bodies unable to digest gluten, a protein found in wheat, barley, and rye. An estimated 5 percent of the population have some degree of gluten intolerance, which can trigger the symptoms of celiac disease: bloating, fatigue, headaches, gastrointestinal issues. Yet one survey of competitive endurance athletes found that 40 percent of them avoid gluten.

Of course some people have food sensitivities. You might produce more mucus after consuming a given

amount of dairy than someone else. That's different from an allergy, however, and might not warrant avoiding dairy altogether. It's also worth investigating whether you really have a sensitiv-

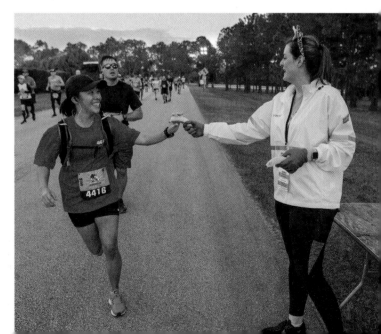

ity or intolerance toward a type of food. For example, you might experience bloating after eating grain products not because of the gluten but because of the fiber in those products. The bottom line: before you decide to avoid a food group for health reasons, work with a nutritionist to determine what's really going on.

Go easy on processed foods. (Sorry, they don't count as one of the major food groups.) We're all busy; cooking from scratch daily isn't realistic for many people. But ask yourself this when thinking about a given food: If I had the time, desire, and cooking chops, could I reasonably make this at home? Can I even pronounce all the ingredients?

Prepared items such as a chicken Caesar salad or Asian noodle bowl pass this test much more so than things like hot dogs and chips.

You might find yourself naturally gravitating toward eating like this as a runner. Some foods that are satisfying in the moment eventually don't seem worth it given how they make you feel on your next run. That's not because running will make you a "health nut" or whatever disparaging term non-runners might throw at you. It's just that, as running becomes more important to you, you realize that there's a difference between the sentiments of "I can eat this" and "I want to eat this."

THE WRONG KIND OF TROTTING

You've probably noticed that running has a way of moving things along in your gastrointestinal system. Overall, that's good. It's believed that quicker food evacuation times is a major reason why runners have lower rates of colon cancer than sedentary people.

But it's not so good when your runs are frequently interrupted by pit stops. Having runner's trots can be annoying (especially to your running partners), embarrassing, even disastrous, if you're on pace for a personal best but lose time in a porta-john.

If you have to take a lot of bathroom breaks while

running, you'll want to do some detective work. Look for patterns in how what you eat ties in to the frequency of pit stops made during a run. Focus on one culprit at a time (or class of culprit, on the reasonable grounds that if a black bean burrito for lunch causes problems on a post-work run, then a pinto bean burrito probably will, too).

If what you eat doesn't seem to matter, then experiment with when you eat. There's great variability among runners when it comes to stomach sensitivity. Some can eat pretty much anything up until starting their run, while others would do best to avoid any food for

a few hours before running. You're probably somewhere in between. Once you've established when is too soon to eat before you run, plan accordingly. It's better to alter your eating schedule a little than to once again find yourself looking for the nearest bushes.

With both content and timing of food intake, be more conservative if you're planning to run fast, long, or in hot weather. These choices and conditions will result in more blood being diverted from your gastrointestinal system to help with the demands of running.

SHOULD YOU TAKE DIETARY SUPPLEMENTS?

The principle that there's no one magic food that will make you a better runner also extends to supplements. There's no evidence that taking, say, three times more than the recommended amount of a given vitamin or mineral will give you three times the benefit. Your body will use what it needs and discard the rest; the primary result you'll get from megadoses of vitamins and minerals is expensive urine.

Many runners take a daily multivitamin. They do so as a form of insurance to ensure they're not deficient when it comes to a key vitamin or mineral. There's no real harm in this better-safe-than-sorry approach, because most multivitamins contain moderate amounts of their ingredients.

But don't lean on multivitamins to make up for not eating a well-balanced diet. It's always better to get vitamins and minerals from real food. An orange isn't just a vehicle for delivering vitamin

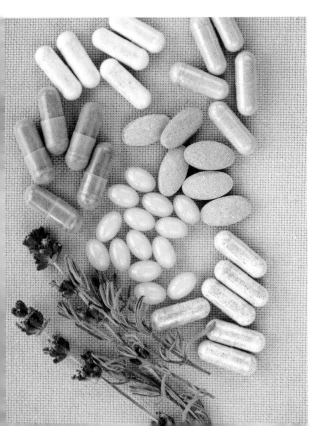

C, nor is a banana a potassium pill that grows on a tree. Real foods contain fiber, phytonutrients (plant chemicals believed to reduce your risk of many chronic diseases), and other beneficial components. These components evolved to work together in a $2 + 2 = 5$ way that manufactured pills can't.

You should be able to meet your vitamin and mineral needs through your diet. A potential exception is vitamin D during the winter. Vitamin D is well known for its role in bone health, but it's also increasingly recognized as a key player in maintaining the immune system.

For most of the year, it's easy to meet your vitamin D needs from a combination of sunlight and diet. Just fifteen minutes of midday sun provides 80 percent of the recommended daily amount from spring through fall in most of North America.

Things change, however, in the winter. You're probably indoors for the bulk of the daylight hours. Also, the sun's ultraviolet B rays transmit much less vitamin D in winter. Compounding the problem is that even when you do run during daylight hours in the winter, you might be clad in gear head to toe because of the cold. Studies have found that people who are low on vitamin D, but not technically deficient, catch more colds and flus during the winter. That's not something you need as a runner, especially with the bulk of runDisney events held January through April.

It can be difficult to meet all of your vitamin D needs through food. Four hard-boiled eggs contain just more than the recommended daily amount of 1,000 international units (IU). Given these challenges, many experts now advise taking a vitamin D supplement from late fall through early spring for people who can't meet their needs from sunlight. As with meeting your needs for other vitamins and minerals, more isn't better. A 1,000 IU vitamin D supplement should suffice.

HANDLING HYDRATION

Here's the short version of how runners should approach hydration: drink to thirst.

If that sounds too simple, then you may have been swayed by well-meaning claims that any degree of dehydration will make you slower, or that everyone should drink eight glasses of water a day. Both claims are incorrect. "Drink to thirst" is the most important thing to remember for staying hydrated throughout the day and when running.

There's no doubt that you want to avoid dehydration. On a run, losing more than 2 percent of your body weight through sweat can force you to slow down. (Less blood returns to your heart, so your heart pumps less blood with each beat, and less oxygen reaches your muscles.) In between runs, being dehydrated can slow your recovery, because waste products aren't removed as quickly, and nutrients that get your body back to normal aren't delivered as rapidly. And you'll just feel bad—you'll have a headache, find it difficult to focus, and be irritable and tired.

But dehydration that interferes with your running and workaday life isn't the same as having sweated. Performance starts to suffer only after you've lost at least 2 percent of your body weight. For a 150-pound person, that's three pounds, or forty-eight ounces of sweat. That's more than most people sweat during normal runs in moderate temperatures. You can probably see why the eight-glasses-of-water-a-day recommendation can't be universally applicable. People of different sizes and activity levels, living in different climates, and perspire at various rates will have differing feelings when it involves thirst.

There's a difference between staying adequately hydrated and always being as hydrated as possible. Drink more than your body needs, and you'll just spend more time looking for the nearest bathroom. If you're adequately hydrated, you won't be thirsty, and your urine will be a pale yellow, similar to the color of straw. So, if you're thirsty or

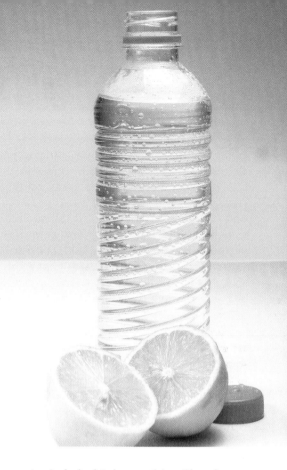

your urine is dark, drink something. If you're not thirsty or your urine is clear, don't drink. It's that simple!

You're more likely to stay properly hydrated by drinking smaller amounts more frequently than doing a couple of camel-at-the-oasis chug sessions per day. It's a good idea at work or when traveling to always have a bottle handy. That's especially true when you're running in hot weather, and being vigilant about your thirst can be more challenging. You don't want to find yourself with a run coming up feeling parched. That means you'll start your run dehydrated, and might sooner have to slow your pace.

While water should be your most frequent beverage, other liquids count toward your hydration needs. The thought used to be that coffee and other caffeinated beverages had a diuretic effect (aka having to pee more) and dehydrated you; the belief was that you had to take in extra fluids then

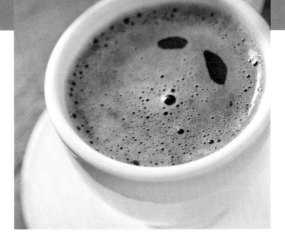

to make up for them. But it's now known that if you regularly drink caffeinated beverages, over twenty-four hours, they don't dehydrate you. The extra urination that occurs in the few hours after you drink them is countered by less urination later. (For more on coffee and running, see "Enjoy Your Coffee!")

What about on the run? "Drink to thirst" remains your guide. In studies where runners on treadmills have easy access to fluids and are told to drink whenever they want, they tend to drink enough to finish just below that 2-percent-of-body-weight threshold.

These studies usually involve longer runs (ninety minutes or more) done in warm to hot conditions. It's unlikely you'll get dehydrated enough to start to feel thirsty on a typical hour-or-shorter run in moderate conditions. So, don't worry about carrying a bottle on most of your runs unless you live where you're going to sweat buckets during a standard run.

Drinking to thirst during a run gets a little trickier when you run long or hard, or the heat and humidity are high, or there's some combination of these factors. If you want to truly tend to your thirst, you'll need to carry fluids or plan routes with easy access to them (bottles you've stashed, or a water fountain, or a convenience store, in close proximity).

Getting dehydrated a little past 2 percent of your body weight isn't dangerous. Whether you want to take steps to avoid that threshold is up to you. If you don't mind slowing a little but do

ENJOY YOUR COFFEE!

Running and coffee are inseparable . . . and for good reason. Many studies have found that caffeine can improve endurance performances. This is thought to happen primarily because caffeine stimulates your central nervous system (as you may have noticed). That stimulation can make a given pace feel easier to maintain, meaning either you can sustain that pace for longer, or you can run slightly faster and still be at a manageable effort level. Coffee drinking is also associated with health benefits such as lower rates of diabetes, heart disease, and depression.

Coffee, though, can interfere with your running by triggering headaches, touching off feelings of being "on the edge," and causing stomach problems, which may lead to on-the-run pit stops. To mitigate such possibilities, experiment to find out the amount you can drink and the timing that works best for you pre-run. Some early-morning runners can sip coffee on the way out the door. Others who are more sensitive have learned to allow enough time for the coffee to provoke a pre-run bathroom trip. If you're in the latter group, make good use of that extra time by doing a full pre-run stretching routine.

CARRYING YOUR CALORIES

As detailed in "Handling Hydration" (see page 45), you don't need to carry water or sport-nutrition products on your average runs. There's no harm finishing runs a little dehydrated. Carrying a bottle for the sake of a few sips on a four-mile run simply isn't worth the inconvenience for most runners.

Your on-the-go fluid and calorie needs increase the longer you run. Depending on the weather, consider carrying fluids and/or food when you're running for longer than ninety minutes. There are a variety of products for this purpose. The ones that are best for you comes down to what and how much you'll be carrying and where you want to place an item during a run. Some fuel belts have removable or expandable components so that you can downsize your haul on shorter outings or increase capacity when you're going to carry lots of liquid and munchies.

Be sure to settle on a product that has minimal effect on your running form. Some runners swear by fluid backpacks; others find the sacs cause them to hunch forward.

Arm straps for bottles might cause you to run a little lopsided. Even a handheld bottle seems to throw off the gaits of some runners.

If you can't find a comfortable solution that works for you when it comes to carrying liquid and food, there's always the old-school approach of stashing bottles along your route. If you're taking that approach, pockets in your apparel can accommodate whatever solid foods you want to run with.

mind carrying bottles, it's okay to finish with losses of 3 or 4 percent, assuming you make rehydrating your top priority afterward. If your run is a key workout leading up to a race, it's worth the hassle to make sure you don't get too far past that 2 percent threshold. You want to be able to meet the goal of the workout, whether that's covering a certain distance or holding a certain pace.

DO YOU NEED SPORT DRINKS, ENERGY GELS, AND THE LIKE?

Part of the overemphasis on hydration that's become a commonplace theme in the running community comes from the sports-drink providers themselves. Now that you know that you're not going to collapse from being a little (or temporarily) dehydrated, you're ready to have a good perspective on sport-nutrition products.

Most people have no reason to sip sports drinks, energy drinks, etc. throughout the day. Water and other sugar-free beverages will keep you hydrated—and food will meet your energy needs. A quart of a typical sports drink contains about 200 calories, almost all from simple sugars, and few to no significant nutrients. That's not a great bargain for your wallet or body, especially if you're watching your weight. A good diet will also replace the electrolytes (primarily sodium and potassium) lost in sweat during normal runs in non-extreme weather.

There's a better argument for consuming sports drinks while running. Most sport drinks contain 6 to 8 percent carbohydrates. That concentration is absorbed as readily as water, and the carbohydrates can help your performance in runs that last longer than an hour. That infusion helps you maintain a fast pace longer, or run longer before your body's carbohydrate stores are depleted, or by making a given pace feel easier. (Your brain's only fuel source is carbohydrates, so when it feels well-fed, running is more likely to feel doable.) The sodium in sports drinks is useful during runs because it helps with water and glucose absorption.

Gels and other easily carried sport-nutrition products are a convenient way to take in calories on the run without having to constantly drink. Most energy gels contain about 100 calories, roughly the amount of energy needed to cover a mile. Having a gel every hour or so on long runs should help you comfortably cover more distance, because your body's stores of carbohydrates will last longer. More isn't better, however—your stomach can process these gels only so quickly. It's best to have a gel soon before you'll have access to fluids, to speed absorption.

LOSING WEIGHT AS A RUNNER

If you want to lose weight by combining diet and exercise, congratulations—you've picked the healthiest, safest, most effective way to lose weight and maintain your new weight long-term.

Note the phrase "long-term." It's relatively easy to lose weight over a short period, especially if you're willing to go to extremes and jeopardize your health. But the same principle we looked at in chapter 2 concerning improving your speed and endurance applies here—*hurry slowly.* Remember that you didn't get to your current weight overnight. Make a plan that systematically helps you reach your goal and is sustainable. Crash dieting is no more effective than crash training, and is perhaps even worse for you.

Along those lines, focus on overall trends. Don't place too much emphasis on daily weigh-ins, just like you shouldn't draw grand conclusions about your fitness from any one run. Your weight can fluctuate significantly even over the course of a day. As long as things are moving in the right direction, you're doing great.

What diet should you follow? Your best bet for long-term success is to follow the broad outlines described earlier of what makes a good diet for all runners. If you eat smaller portions while running enough to achieve a modest calorie deficit most days, you'll eventually lose weight. Eating to lose weight can be a great time to refocus on the quality of your diet. If you're eating less than usual, then you want everything you eat to be that much more nutrient-dense.

A daily deficit of 500 more calories expended than consumed will result in the loss of about one pound a week. A mile of walking or running burns approximately 100 calories. So, if you want to create a weekly deficit of 3,500 calories to lose a pound, and run fifteen miles a week, that leaves 2,000 calories total over the week, or less than 300 a day, to eat less of.

You've probably heard people say weight loss isn't as simple as calories in, calories out. You can also find people who split hairs over whether running burns more calories per mile than walking, or who get hung up on differences in calories burned per mile between a twenty-five-year-old who weighs 150 pounds and a fifty-five-year-old who weighs 180. There are differences in efficiency, metabolism, and other factors that can affect the precise numbers. But for the hurry-slow, long-term approach, it really does come down to calories in versus calories out.

It's quite possible to train for a race while cutting back a little on food. The key is to make sure you're adequately fueled for your longest and other most important runs. It's better for your race and your weight-loss goal to have eaten enough to get through your main runs strongly. Just as your running mileage varies throughout the week, so can your caloric intake.

Your appetite will usually be suppressed for a while after you run, especially in warmer weather. Once that feeling subsides, avoid two common mistakes. First, don't overeat because you've "earned it." If your normal run is five miles but instead you went eight, nice going. But remember that in doing so you burned an additional 300 calories. That extra amount is easily made up and then some if you down a huge breakfast or even just an extra doughnut.

Second, don't wait so long to eat after running to the point that you develop "runger." Going too long without calories after you run can lead to overcompensating later. In general, while slight hunger pangs are common when you're losing weight, don't allow yourself to get ravenous. Eat often enough that you're never truly famished and at risk of undoing several days' worth of good work.

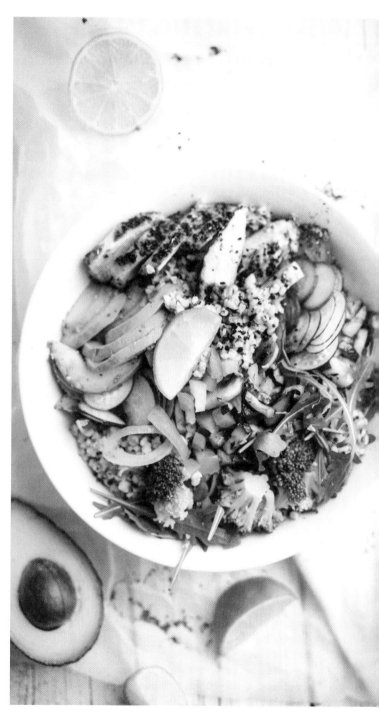

THE MYTH OF THE FAT-BURNING ZONE

You may have heard about working out in a special fat-burning zone to accelerate weight loss. The best thing to do with this claim: ignore it. Focus on *calories in, calories out.*

The longer explanation of why not to get fixated on the fat-burning-zone myth requires some detail. First, the claim: exercising in a low-intensity zone of about 60 percent of your maximal heart rate will burn more fat than if you run (or bike, or ski, etc.) the same distance at a higher intensity. In running terms, the supposed fat-burning zone corresponds to a gentle jog at which you could easily converse in complete sentences.

It's true that running at this leisurely pace burns more fat than doing the same distance faster. When you run, you burn a mixture of carbohydrates (stored in your muscles as glycogen) and fat (stored, well, you know). Fat requires a lot of oxygen to burn. It's extremely inefficient to burn that fat when oxygen is scarce, as is the case when you're running fast. So, the faster you go, the higher the percentage of the carb-fat fuel mix that's supplied by carbohydrates; the slower you go, the higher the percentage of that fuel mix that's supplied by fat. Therefore, the claim goes, slow down, and you'll burn more fat.

Perhaps you can see the problem with this logic. At rest, about 85 percent of your energy needs are met by burning fat. If you stand up and walk across the room, you'll start burning a little more carbohydrate and a little less fat. Pick up the pace of your walk, and you'll burn even less fat. By no means should you break into a run, because then you'll be burning even less fat. If all that matters is what percentage of your fuel mix is supplied by fat, then you should spend all of your time sitting or lying in bed . . . because you'll really be in the fat-burning zone!

A less facetious explanation goes like this: First, the difference in total fat burned in running three miles slowly and doing the same distance faster is perhaps a couple dozen calories. That's negligible in the grand scheme of things, given that burning a pound of fat entails burning about 3,500 calories. It's not as if working out in the supposed fat-burning zone magically sucks fat out of wherever you wish you didn't have it.

More important, focusing on the percentage of calories burned from fat ignores that calories in—calories out remains the true basis of weight loss. You could spend an hour walking three miles, and of the roughly 300 calories you'd burn, a higher percentage would be from fat than if you ran three miles. But in that hour, you could run five or more miles, burning more than 500 calories (and an overall greater number of calories from fat, if you really want to get geeky over the math). In addition, your metabolism stays revved up longer after vigorous workouts than it does after exercising at the low-intensity level associated with the fat-burning zone.

The takeaway, once again, is this: focus on *calories in, calories out.* Use the rough figure of 100 calories per mile covered on foot. Yes, there are slight differences based on body size, genetics, fitness level, and other factors. But these differences are splitting hairs compared to the overall burn-more-calories-than-you-consume reality.

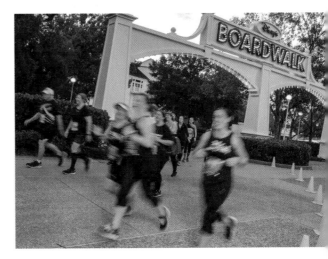

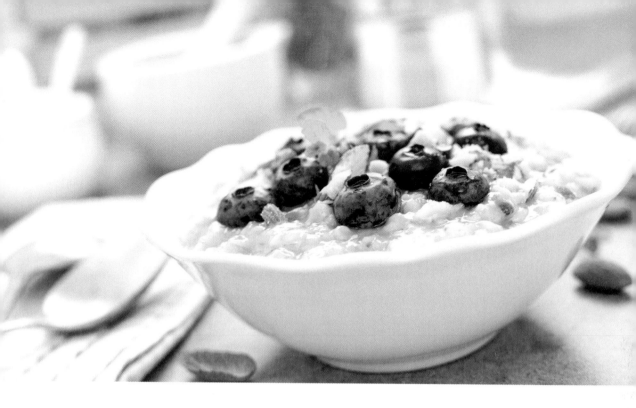

RACE-DAY NUTRITION

Many runners worry too much about what to eat the day before and on the day of a race.

No great changes are necessary—or advisable—to your regular diet. For most races, enjoy a normal dinner the night before. There's no need to emphasize extra carbohydrates before races shorter than a half marathon. Lean toward blander food and avoid large amounts of high-fiber foods, such as beans and cruciferous vegetables, to reduce your chances of gastrointestinal problems the next day. But otherwise, eat a sensible amount of foods you enjoy and are accustomed to. Drink enough water to be adequately hydrated, using thirst and the color of your urine as guides.

Before a half marathon or longer race, eat carbohydrate-rich meals throughout the preceding day so that your muscles are stocked with the fuel you'll burn on race day. That's a better approach than eating nonchalantly the first part of the day and then sitting down to a massive plate of pasta. Eating a large, excessive dinner won't

lead to you storing as many carbohydrates as eating a good amount of carbohydrates throughout the day. You're also less likely to have digestion issues with smaller, more frequent carb-rich meals.

Ideally, you'll have found what works for you in terms of pre-run nutrition before your longest training runs. Before heading into a race that's shorter than a half marathon, you're fine not eating breakfast on race day if that's what you're used to. On the morning of a half marathon or one that's longer, try eating a few hundred calories (a banana and half a bagel, or maybe oatmeal with a banana) two to three hours before the start. Yes, this will mean getting up that much earlier. The trade-off of having topped-off fuel stores is usually worth it.

Continue to hydrate using the drink-to-thirst guidance. Sipping a sports drink before the start will hydrate you as well as water, and it will provide you with a little extra energy for races of a half marathon or longer.

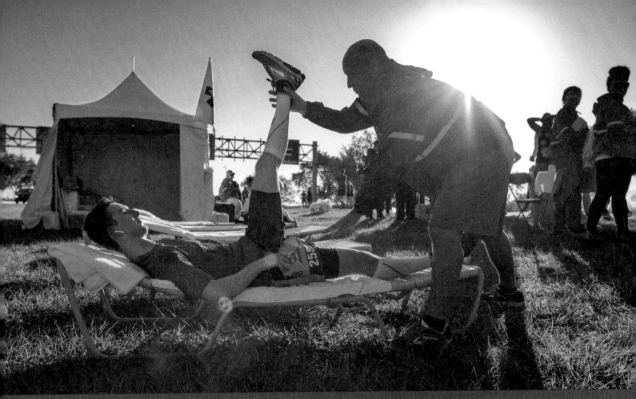

CHAPTER 5:
HOW TO PREVENT AND TREAT COMMON RUNNING INJURIES

Here's a time-saver for you: don't Google "How Many Runners Get Injured." You'll see a wide range of stats, with claims that somewhere between 25 percent and 90 percent (!) of runners get injured every year.

The reason not to search this topic isn't because runners don't get hurt. We do. But these estimates are not presented in the proper context. How is *injury* defined? Something that hurts but that doesn't keep you from running? Something that's fine if you take two days off? Two weeks off? More important, why did each of the runners surveyed get injured?

These are important questions, because without knowing the answers to them, it's easy to think that being a runner means you're going to

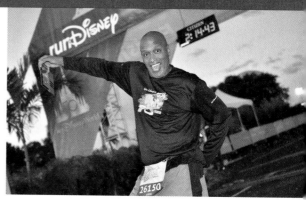

spend much of your time injured. That's a fatalistic view. The better perspective is that you have the power to keep most running injuries at bay. In this chapter, we'll look at how you do this, as well as how to overcome common injuries if you do wind up with one. It's the longest chapter in the book, because remaining as injury-free as possible underlies all success and enjoyment in running.

WHAT ARE RUNNING INJURIES?

Let's start by understanding the nature of most running injuries. Sure, you might get hurt from slipping on the ice or tripping on the trail, or taking too wonky a step while trying to sidestep an unleashed dog. But those acute, dramatic injuries are the exception, akin to incidents from your life outside running that keep you from running, such as wrenching your lower back while cleaning out the attic.

Almost all running injuries are overuse injuries, or what sports medicine professionals call repetitive strain injuries. A vulnerable body part can no longer handle the low-grade but repeated stress of running, and says enough is enough. A tendon swells with inflammation. A muscle gets a micro-tear. A bone develops an ever-so-slight fracture.

That might sound as if running injuries are inevitable. They're not. And that's good news! That means you can do something to prevent them, and if you get injured, you can do something to keep them from happening again.

Think about running injuries like an engineer would: some part of your structure couldn't withstand the pressure it was under. If an engineer were examining a vulnerable bridge, she would have two main concerns: how to lessen the strain on the structure, and how to strengthen the structure. The same approach applies to avoiding running injuries.

RUNNING SHOES AND INJURY

You'll remember from chapter 3 that running shoes can't prevent injuries. But they can lower your risk of getting hurt. The right shoes will work with rather than against your body. When you're in shoes that feel like an extension of your feet, you'll run with better form, and thereby lessen the strain on your body. Running shoes that match your unique makeup will engage your strongest body parts and not put too much of the stress of running on your weaker parts.

TWO KEYS TO AVOIDING INJURY

Good training and a good running body are your two main bulwarks against getting a running injury. Let's look in detail at what both of these broad concepts mean.

Good training in regard to injury more or less mirrors good training in regard to performance. Avoid doing too much, too soon, and too hard. We saw in chapters 1 and 2 how to safely increase your mileage. Following those principles will help you avoid the "too much" and "too soon" traps.

"Too hard" doesn't mean to do only slow running. As we'll see, regularly running at a variety of paces is likely to lower, not increase, your injury risk chances. Instead, "too hard" means that you feel like you're always pushing, in terms of distance, pace, or both. If you spend the second half of most of your runs wishing you were done, you're too often working too hard. You should finish most runs feeling energized, not exhausted. In your last mile or two, ask yourself whether you could keep going for at least another mile at your current effort level. Most days, the answer should be *yes*.

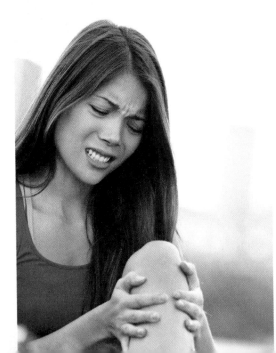

These are admittedly broad, subjective guidelines. What "too much, too soon, too hard" mean together varies greatly by individual. You might need three recovery days after your longest runs, while your training partner might feel fully recovered after two. Similarly, some people can handle upping their mileage by 20 percent per week, while others get hurt when they attempt much smaller increases. Figuring out your unique thresholds for these factors is key to putting together what "good training" is for you. A detailed training log is invaluable in this regard. Your log can reveal patterns in how you handle various mixes of mileage and intensity.

It's always better to be a little under-trained than a little overtrained. That's true when you're building toward a race, because when you get too fatigued over a period of time, you can't absorb the benefits of your hard work, and you stagnate or get slower. It's especially true for injury-avoidance purposes. Pushing that last 1 or 2 percent will get you, at best, only marginally fitter, yet will increase your injury risk significantly. Which sounds more satisfying: being 95 percent fit and uninjured, or being unable to run because you asked your body to do more than it was capable of? The first goal of any race-training program should be to get you to the start line healthy.

It's typical to realize you've overstepped your body's current capacity only once it's too late. You feel a little calf tightness with two miles to go but carry on, and by the next day you can't walk normally. Or you feel out of whack but stick with your long-run plan, because you don't want to be a wimp—and consequently wind up with a hitch in your hip that costs you a week of running. Older runners (say, forty and over) in particular can't afford these kinds of mistakes. What when we were in our twenties might have been slight flare-ups that "heal" in a day or two can become chronic, low-grade annoyances once we're older and our bodies don't recover like they used to.

VARY VERY MUCH

Much of the just-noted circumstances ties into not overstressing your body in terms of distance. Another way to lower the stress of running on your body is to vary that stress. There are two key ways to do this. First, vary the elements of your training. In the first two chapters, we looked at the basic parts of a well-rounded training program. The emphasis in those chapters was on how having a mixture of shorter and longer runs—and easier and harder runs—builds your fitness better than doing the same type of run every day. Well, it turns out that having variety in your training should also lower your injury risk.

Running at a variety of paces means you'll use a slightly different stride most days. Many people assume that running faster will increase their injury risk. But if you warm up properly and don't overextend yourself, short bouts of faster running will usually have you running taller and landing and pushing off more toward the front of your foot than when you run at an easy pace. Your body will appreciate the slight shift in dynamics. In addition, faster running engages muscles a little differently than slower running, and can help to build muscular strength. All of this means your body will experience whatever your weekly mileage is differently than if you run the same pace all the time.

Similarly, running a variety of distances means that some days are relatively easier on your body. If you've

built up to handling longer runs properly, a twenty-five-mile week consisting of one ten-mile run, a seven-mile run, and two four-mile runs should place less repetitive strain on your weakest parts than a week consisting of five five-mile runs.

It's also helpful to vary the topography and terrain of your runs. Running a flat course some days and a hillier one on other days will engage slightly different muscles. Mixing up the surfaces you run on changes the nature of the impact force your body absorbs. Many runners gravitate to softer surfaces instinctively, because they feel less beat up after running on dirt than if they do most of their running on asphalt or cement. It's not uncommon for runners who have access to trails during the warmer months to feel achier and creakier in the winter, when trails are unavailable and they have to do all of their running on the roads.

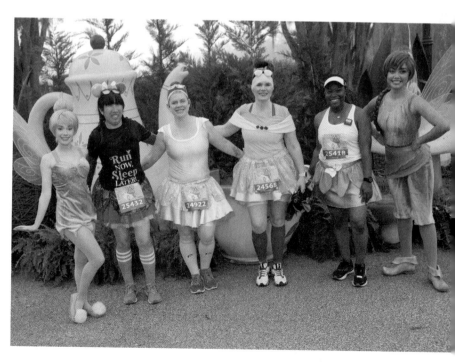

NO, RUNNING WON'T RUIN YOUR KNEES

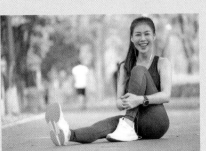

You'll know you've arrived as a runner when you get your first lecture on how you're going to destroy your knees. This "advice" is usually based on the belief that running increases your risk of developing osteoarthritis in your knees. It doesn't.

Here are the facts: Numerous studies have shown that runners (and other regular exercisers) have lower rates of knee osteoarthritis than sedentary people. For example, a study published in 2008 in the *American Journal of Preventive Medicine* followed runners and non-runners for almost twenty years. X-rays showed signs of arthritis in the knees of 20 percent of the runners, but 32 percent in those of non-runners.

A potential counterargument against such findings is that when the studies commence, the longtime runners that take part have above-average structural health—that they don't include people who started running but had to give it up because their bodies broke down.

Research, however, has rebutted that stance as well. A study published in 2017 in *Arthritis Care Research* followed more than two thousand people for several years to see how many developed arthritic knees. The participants gave detailed information on how often they had knee pain and its severity. They also described their current and former exercise habits. In other words, the participants weren't selected because of whether they were or weren't runners.

But it turned out that their running status did matter. Regarding frequency of knee pain, symptoms of arthritis, and evidence of arthritis shown in x-rays, current runners had significantly better scores than non-runners. For example, current runners were 29 percent less likely than non-runners to report frequent knee pain. Even former runners were less likely to report knee pain and show signs of arthritis than non-runners. That last finding is the opposite of what should

be the case if running ruined their knees and caused them to give up the sport.

Why might runners have lower rates of knee arthritis? First, runners tend to have a lower body mass index than average people. Less excess weight means less strain on your joints, including your knees. Second, many experts believe that running has an anti-inflammatory effect on joints. Think of increased circulation of synovial fluid as lubrication for the knees. Sedentary people who have developed osteoarthritis are advised to exercise regularly for these exact reasons.

The takeaway: yes, some runners get arthritis in their knees. But all available evidence indicates they do so at a significantly lower rate than non-runners. Therefore, it's reasonable to conclude that something besides running is the underlying cause.

HOW CROSS-TRAINING CAN LOWER YOUR INJURY RISK

Cross-training is another way to reduce—or more accurately, remove—the impact forces of running. If you struggle to stay healthy while trying to reach a certain level of mileage, one or two days per week of cross-training can advance your overall fitness while giving your body a break from the pounding. Cross-training can also bring many of the benefits you enjoy from running, such as weight control, a chance to socialize, time in nature, and the simple pleasure of the activity itself.

Cross-training here means aerobic exercise—swimming, cycling, Nordic skiing, and other activities where you sustain an elevated heart rate for twenty or more minutes. Non-aerobic activities such as yoga and resistance training will definitely help your running as well. But consider them supplementary activities that you engage in to complement your running, not to replace it on some days.

And sorry, but doing something like working in the garden or raking leaves isn't cross-training. They're just things you do as a healthy person living a full life.

Obviously, you need to run enough to be able to meet the goals you've set. Running a half marathon or longer will not be a magical experience if your body isn't mechanically prepared to go the distance, no matter how good your cardiovascular fitness is. Cross-training is best considered for injury avoidance by swapping it for some of your shorter runs. A great time to schedule cross-training for this purpose is on the day after your longest and/or hardest runs. It's on those days, rather than while doing the actual challenging run, that you're most likely to feel exhausted and find it difficult to run with good form.

What type of cross-training is best for runners? The kind that you're most likely to do most often. If you love to swim but the nearest pool is a forty-minute drive away, and the pool has lap swimming only between 6 a.m. and 7:30 a.m., you're probably better off finding an alternative option. Or maybe you live two minutes from a spin bike facility, but absolutely hate stationary cycling. It's probably going to be tough then to attend enough sessions to help your running. Experiment with different activities to find one you enjoy (or at least tolerate) and that's realistically doable around everything else going on in your life. If more than one type of cross-training activity meets these criteria, all the better.

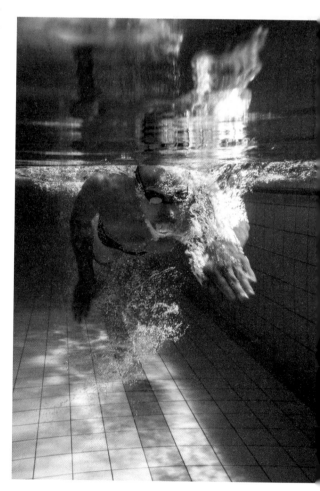

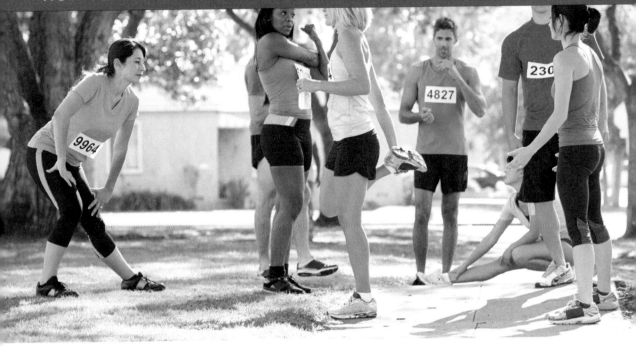

BUILDING A BETTER RUNNING BODY

So far, we've looked at how to lessen running's repetitive strain on your body. But that's only half of the injury-avoidance equation. The other part: make the structure better able to withstand the repetitive strain.

To understand this idea, consider runners you might think are impervious to injury—high schoolers. Teenage runners actually get injured quite frequently. The reason is, as a leading high school coach puts it, "Their engine is more advanced than their chassis." That is, their cardiovascular system (the engine) allows them to run at a volume and intensity that their bones, ligaments, muscles, and tendons (the chassis) aren't yet able to handle. Those same runners often have fewer injuries in college, however, even though they're training harder; their bodies have grown more capable of absorbing the pounding.

Adult runners, of course, have fully grown skeletons. Where our structure often suffers is with its alignment and connective materials. Years of sitting and otherwise being subject to gravity can throw us out of balance. If we've been sedentary for much of our adult lives, our muscles tend to be short, tight, and weak. Extra weight increases the load on our joints. Even if we've stayed active, we probably don't regularly move through a wide range of motion in all directions. We've settled into movement patterns that accommodate our areas of greatest tightness and weakness.

This process feeds on itself, so that we feel constrained or restricted when we try to break out of those patterns. When we run, one or more body parts aren't strong and/or flexible enough to handle the repetitive stress they're under. So, either they start to break down, or our bodies shift the load to other body parts that are asked to take on more than they're meant to handle. And then we're injured.

So, let's improve our structure! Even runners who have never been injured don't say, "I sure wish I were weaker and tighter."

THINK *PREHAB*, NOT REHAB

The good news is that increasing your resistance to running injury is usually simple and straightforward. A small amount of work a few days a week can go a long way.

It's common for injured runners to be dedicated to their rehab exercises, and then ditch those exercises when they're pain-free. It's also common for those runners to get hurt again, and start the injury/rehab/gradually-resume-running cycle anew.

What's better is to consider strengthening and stretching exercises a fundamental part of your running, rather than something you do only when you're injured. The idea here is to prevent problems from happening, rather than waiting for them to develop. Think of spending a few minutes a day on bettering your running body as insurance. It's a small price to pay for the ability to run like you want to and to feel good doing so.

The best way to regularly do "prehab" work is to sandwich your runs with exercises. Coming up is a basic pre- and post-run routine that will increase your running-specific strength and flexibility; no equipment is required. When planning your runs, include the time it will take to do these exercises. That approach will result in more consistency than if you tell yourself you'll do the exercises when you have the time. Plus, doing these few exercises around your runs will help you feel better when you start that day's run, and set you up to feel better on your next run.

If you already have (or get recommended) a more individualized, more ambitious pre- and post-run routine, great—go for it! Here's an excellent start, though, if you don't. As with running regularly, first establish the habit of doing prehab exercises, and then think about going beyond the basics.

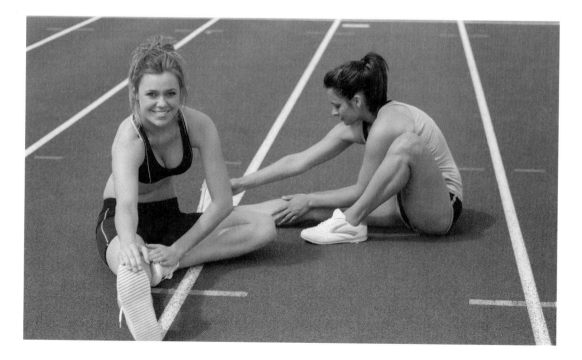

A SHORT, SIMPLE PRE-RUN ROUTINE

These exercises will increase circulation, warm your muscles, loosen your joints, and set your body up to run with good form from your first step. Repeat each exercise ten times before starting the next one. (For the ones that work one leg at a time, do ten on each side.)

CAT-COW: Get in a table position, with your feet, knees, and palms on the floor. Inhale and gently arch your back while looking up slightly. Hold for a few seconds. Exhale while pulling in your abs to round your back and tucking your chin to your chest. Return to the start position. Increase the degree of both stretches as your pelvic area and lower back loosen up.

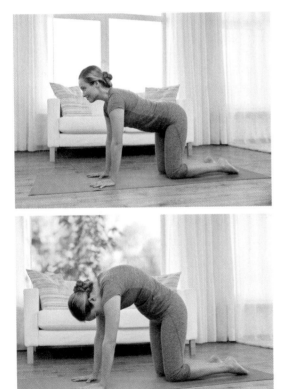

The two phases of cat-cow stretch.

BIRD DOG: Get in a table position. Extend your right arm and left leg straight while keeping your hips level. Return to table position, and repeat on the other side.

BRIDGES: Lie on your back with your feet flat on the floor and your arms at your sides. Push your hips up by engaging your glutes, and return to the start position. Don't use your arms to push up.

SIDE LEG SWINGS: Stand with your arms straight out and against a wall or a raised surface that's at least waist-high. While keeping it straight and just in front of your left leg, swing your right leg to the side and then across your body. Gently increase your range of motion with each swing.

FRONT LEG SWINGS: Stand with your right hand braced against a table, countertop, or other surface that's about waist-high. Keeping it straight, swing your right leg in front of you. Gently increase your range of motion with each swing. Turn around and place your left hand on the surface, and repeat with your left leg.

WALK KNEE TO CHEST: While standing tall, grab your right knee with both hands. Bring it to your chest primarily by lifting your leg and pressing down firmly with your left foot. At the top of the movement, use your hands to lift the leg a little higher. As you return your right foot to a neutral standing position, begin the same knee-to-chest movement with your left leg.

WALK FOOT TO BUTT: While standing tall, use your right hand to grab your right foot and pull it toward your butt. At the same time, press down firmly through your left foot while reaching high with your left arm. As you return your right foot to a neutral standing position, begin the same foot-to-butt movement with your left leg.

A SHORT, SIMPLE POST-RUN ROUTINE

You may have noticed that none of the pre-run exercises are conventional static stretches, where you assume a position that stretches a muscle and then hold that position for several seconds. That's because active stretches like those just cited are better than static stretches for warming up when your muscles are cold. After running, once your muscles are warm, is the time to work on your flexibility.

The post-run routine starts with some soothing static stretches. Hold each for thirty seconds and perform the stretch once or twice. Then you move into a few basic strengthening exercises that feel best to do when you're still energized from your run.

CALF WALL STRETCH: Stand facing a wall from about an arm's length away. Place your palms on the wall and slide your left foot back so that your weight is on your right foot. Bend your right knee until you feel a gentle stretch in your lower calf muscles. Then straighten your left leg while keeping your right foot flat and your right knee bent. You should now feel a stretch in your upper calf muscles. Repeat on the other side.

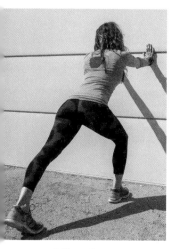

HAMSTRING STRETCH: Lie on your back with your legs straight. While keeping it straight, raise your right leg by contracting your thigh muscles. Lace your hands behind your right leg to gently increase the stretch. If doing this stretch with your left leg straight is too challenging, start over with the sole of your left foot on the floor. Repeat on the other side.

Calf stretch.

HIP FLEXOR STRETCH: Place your right foot flat on the floor in front of you so that your knee is at a ninety-degree angle. Kneel on your left knee, with the knee slightly behind your hips. Stay tall through your spine as you slightly bend your right knee. You should feel a stretch along the front of your left hip. Deepen the stretch by bending your right knee more and/or raising your left arm toward the ceiling. Repeat on the other side.

GLUTE STRETCH: Lie on your back and bring your knees toward your chest. Cross your right knee over your left knee, grab your shins or ankles, and flex your toes toward your shins. Pull your knees closer to your chest while slightly moving your feet away from each other. You should feel a stretch deep in your right glute. Repeat on the other side.

LOWER BACK STRETCH: If you've done yoga, you know child's pose, which is what we'll do here. From a kneeling position, tuck your feet under your lower legs and slowly stack your thighs on top of your lower legs. At the same time, reach out with straight arms as you stack your chest atop your thighs. Place your forehead on the floor. Once you're in the position, concentrate on elongating your back by simultaneously reaching through your fingers and gently moving your butt away from your shoulders.

If your knees or ankles prevent you from comfortably getting into child's pose, try the happy baby pose instead. Lie on your back with your head on the floor and your knees bent toward your chest. Grab your toes or the outside of your feet and gently pull your knees closer to your

Lower back stretch.

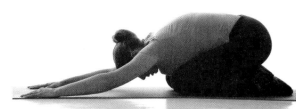

shoulders. Gradually deepen the stretch as you feel your lower back starting to relax.

Now it's time for a little strengthening. These exercises will help you maintain good form when you start to tire on the run. They mostly target the muscles of your shoulders, back, hips, and glutes. It's functional strength in those muscles, rather than six-pack abs, that will keep your trunk stable when you run. Having that stability will lower your risk of sustaining some kind of running injury. Many studies have found a connection between a weak midsection and injury elsewhere, such as the knee; that's because trunk instability is likely to lead to excess or other undesirable motion elsewhere.

Do ten reps on both sides for each leg exercise. For planks, work up to holding each position for thirty seconds. For push-ups and dips, do only as many as you can while maintaining a neutral spine. Over time, try to build up to doing twenty push-ups and twenty dips in your routine.

FIRE HYDRANT: Get in a table position, with your feet, knees, and palms on the floor. Keep your spine neutral. While keeping it bent at ninety degrees, raise your right leg so that your lower leg is parallel to the floor (as if you're a dog marking a fire hydrant). Draw your leg back toward you to the start position.

JANE FONDA: From a table position, use your glutes to raise your right foot behind while keeping your leg bent at ninety degrees. Imagine you're pushing the bottom of your right foot into the ceiling. Return to the start position.

DONKEY KICK: From a table position, keep your right leg bent at ninety degrees while swinging behind you and toward your right shoulder. Imagine that you're trying to hook your toes over your shoulder. Swing the leg back to the start position.

CLAMSHELL: Lie on your left side with your back straight and your right leg stacked over your left leg, with your legs at a ninety-degree angle. Hold your arms together straight in front of you. Using your right glute muscles, pull your bent right leg away from your left leg as far as you can, then slowly bring your right leg back to the start position. Imagine your legs are a clamshell opening and closing.

THREE-WAY LEG RAISE: Lie on your left side with your head, shoulders, hips, and feet aligned. While keeping your right foot parallel to the floor, raise your right leg as high as you comfortably can. Do ten reps with your foot in this position.

Next, do ten leg raises from the same position but with the toes of your right foot pointed toward the ceiling. Then do ten leg raises from the same position with the toes of your right foot pointed toward the floor. Finally, switch to lying on your right side, and repeat the three leg-raise variations with your left leg.

PRONE PLANK: Lie facedown with your weight on your toes and forearms. Keep your elbows in line with your shoulders, your head in line with your hips, and your gaze down. Keep a neutral spine—don't arch your back or raise your butt.

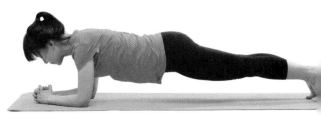

Prone plank.

SUPINE PLANK: Lie faceup with your weight on your heels and forearms. Keep your head, shoulders, and hips aligned. Don't arch your back or allow your hips to sag.

SIDE PLANK: Lie on your right side with your left leg stacked over your right leg and your right forearm at a ninety-degree angle to your body. Raise yourself up so your weight is on the outside of your right foot and your right forearm. Raise your left arm straight into the air while keeping your shoulders squared. Concentrate on maintaining a straight line from your shoulders through your hips—and don't allow your hips to rise or sag. Switch to your left side and repeat.

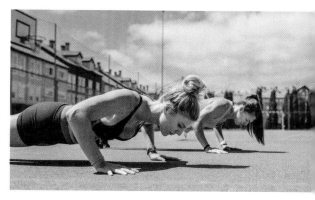

Push-ups.

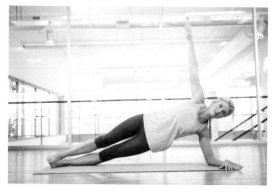

Side plank.

PUSH-UPS: Start facedown with your toes anchored on the floor, your arms straight, and your hands flat on the floor slightly wider than shoulder-width apart as being shown above. Bend

your elbows to lower your body until your chest is just above the floor, then push back up to the start position.

Throughout this routine, keep your hips in line with your shoulders and ankles, and keep your elbows close to your body.

DIP: While facing away from the surface, place your hands on a chair or on another stable surface that's between knee- and waist-height. Your feet should be flat on the floor and your hips should be as close as possible to the raised surface. Bend your elbows to lower your hips toward the floor, then push back up to the start position.

ROLL WITH IT

A foam roller is a great tool to incorporate into routine, both before and after your run. Gently rolling your calves, hamstrings, and hips, as well as along the outside of your thighs before you run, will increase circulation and slightly activate your nervous system, meaning you'll start your runs feeling looser and livelier.

After your run, rolling where you feel tightness will increase blood flow to those areas, lessening the chance of developing a chronic knot in those spots. Many runners shared that they also enjoy a few minutes of foam rolling before going to sleep. Presleep is a great time to roll your upper back and shoulders. Doing so works out the kinks of a busy day and helps you head to bed refreshed.

A FEW OTHER KEYS TO STAYING INJURY-FREE

How you spend your time when not running also affects whether you'll get injured. You don't need to be obsessive and run everything through a how-will-this-affect-my-running filter. But a little mindfulness during the many hours per week you're not running can pay big dividends.

WATCH YOUR POSTURE: Let's be honest: a lot of us are slouchers. Literally. We spend our time hunched over phones and in front of other screens. We slump into our car seats. We binge-watch while half sitting/half reclining as if we're in a hospital bed.

As a result, our default posture strays from the ideal. When we stand, our lower back is flat, our chest is sunken, our shoulders are stooped, and our head is thrust forward. Over time, our hamstrings and glutes tighten and weaken, the hip flexors along the front of our legs shorten, and our neck, shoulders, and head are in a state of permanent tension.

And guess what? We tend to run that way, too. Watch children at a fun run or on an athletic field, and then watch average adults out for their runs, and you'll see a striking difference. (Well, that is at least until kids are about thirteen and have also started spending too much time in that modern-life slouch pose.)

Back in chapter 1, we looked at the basic principles of good running form. When you're not running, try to implement the same basic idea of keeping body parts in alignment. When you're standing or walking, balance your weight evenly between your feet, and keep your head, shoulders, and hips aligned. When sitting, maintain a slight curve in your lower back, keep your feet flat on the floor, and position your head over your shoulders. Keep screens at eye level.

These practices will make it a lot easier to maintain good form when you run, which, in turn, should lower your injury risk.

MOVE MORE: Even if you have the greatest posture in the world, try not to sit for long stretches without a break. Lots of sitting is always going to weaken your glutes and hamstrings, and tighten your hip flexors. Try to get up and move around at least once an hour if your work situation allows it. Walk the halls, go up and down a couple flights of stairs, stand by your workstation and stretch your shoulders and neck. Really, just do anything but keep sitting!

Some researchers have coined the phrase "active couch potato" to describe people who work out but are otherwise as sedentary as everyone else. Don't be like that. If you can find ways to include regular bouts of non-taxing movement into your days, you'll burn more calories, your blood pressure and cholesterol levels will be healthier, and, for the purposes of this chapter, you'll feel better running. Starting your runs looser and more limber will make it easier to do them with good form from the first step.

WATCH YOUR WEIGHT: Try to stay at a good running weight. That's a different goal than being as light as possible. A good running weight is one at which running usually feels pleasurable—you have a nice flow to your stride, your joints don't feel overburdened, your body parts move in sync. At a good running weight, you'll also feel strong and capable most days, rather than fragile and exhausted.

What that weight will be for you is highly specific, depending on things like the body type you were born with, your age, your propensity to add muscle, your non-running activities, and many other factors. One sign that you're in range of your best running weight is that you don't keep getting hurt. Frequent injuries can mean that you could benefit from losing some weight (back to our lessen-the-strain-on-the-structure idea). But repeated injuries—especially to bones—can also mean you might benefit from gaining a few pounds (back to our strengthen-the-structure principle).

Try to avoid wide swings in your weight. Big changes in your weight add a confusing variable to your body's ability to withstand your running regimen. They're also not good for your health in general.

CHECK YOUR NON-RUNNING SHOES: Some runners pore over all available information on running shoes before selecting a pair. Many of them then give no thought to how the shoes they wear for many hours each day they're not running might affect their body.

High heels have been shown to shorten Achilles tendons and calf muscles. Heels also tip your pelvis forward. The tapered front of many dress shoes squeezes toes into unnatural positions. Shoes made of heavy, stiff materials can transmit more of the impact forces of walking up your legs. None of these developments will help your body when it comes to running.

To the extent your job permits it, wear flat, wide, comfortable shoes that will allow your feet to be in a natural, neutral position. If that's not possible, at least wear those kind of shoes when you're not at work. Going barefoot (or in socks or slippers) around the house gives your feet a break from being confined and may help strengthen your foot muscles.

OVERCOMING THE MOST COMMON RUNNING INJURIES

If, despite your best efforts, you do get an injury from running, there are two phases to dealing with it: First, get over the acute, short-term (let's hope!) period in which the injury interferes with your running. Second, take steps to prevent its recurrence. Here's how to handle those two phases for the most common running injuries.

SHIN SPLINTS

WHAT IT IS: Known to medical professionals as *medial tibial stress syndromes*, shin splints are the most common injury for beginning runners. Shin splints arise when the muscle that attaches to the tibia (shinbone) is under excessive stress. You'll usually feel tenderness and pain in the lower portion of the inner shin. Depending on the severity, you might feel shin splints almost from the start of runs, or the pain might come on more gradually and increase during your run.

SHORT-TERM TREATMENT: Cut back on running to less than whatever distance or duration usually brings on your symptoms. Ice the tender area a few times a day, especially after running. If possible, run on soft surfaces to lower your impact forces.

LONG-TERM PREVENTION: Because shin splints often stem from a lack of running-specific strength and/or poor running form, most runners eventually overcome them simply by becoming more experienced. Avoiding overstriding and otherwise running with good form will more evenly distribute running's impact forces.

RUNNER'S KNEE

WHAT IT IS: Also called patellofemoral syndrome, runner's knee is the most common running injury. Pain develops around the front of the knee because the patella (kneecap) isn't aligning well with the femur (thigh bone) when the knee bends or straightens. Pain is usually absent or mild at the start of runs but increases the longer you stay out. Runner's knee is often felt during non-running hours, especially when you first start moving around after sitting for a while.

SHORT-TERM TREATMENT: Runner's knee can keep coming back if you don't get the initial inflammation under control. It's usually best to avoid running for about a week while icing a few times a day. Don't try to run again until you can move about normally without symptoms.

LONG-TERM PREVENTION: Because runner's knee is caused by an alignment problem, the solution is to improve that alignment. This is most often done by strengthening your quadriceps (thigh muscles) and hips; a stronger midsection leads to more stability when you land. Runner's knee can be worsened by heavy heel striking and/or over-striding. Experiment with increasing your cadence (the number of steps you take per minute when running) by 5 percent. This tweak usually helps runners overcome a tendency to crash into the ground when they land.

ILIOTIBIAL BAND SYNDROME

WHAT IT IS: The iliotibial band (IT band) is a thick band of fascia that runs along the outside of your leg from the hip to the knee. IT band syndrome occurs when the IT band is subjected to excessive stress or friction, usually because of the knee rotating and collapsing inward during running. You'll most often feel discomfort or pain along the outside top of the knee when running. When you're not running, you'll most often notice IT band syndrome when you rise after sitting for a while, descend stairs, or squat below a ninety-degree angle.

SHORT-TERM TREATMENT: Sprint uphill every day! Just kidding. But it is an oddity of IT band syn-drome that you'll usually have more discomfort at a slower pace and when going downhill. If you can run without pain and without altering your form, short, easy runs should be okay. Avoid downhill courses, and try to run on level surfaces, because a slanted surface will put more strain on your IT band. That said, you'll probably be free of IT band syndrome sooner if you take one to two weeks off to reduce the inflammation.

Whether you run or not, foam roll or otherwise massage the bottom section of your IT band (from the knee to about halfway up your thigh). Also ice the outside of your knee.

LONG-TERM PREVENTION: Strengthen your quadriceps, hips, and glutes to provide better stability for your knee. If you're a heavy heel striker, experiment with increasing your steps per minute by 5 percent; doing so should shift some impact forces off the knee. Avoiding canted surfaces is good advice for all runners at all times, but it's especially worth being fastidious about if you've had IT band syndrome.

STRESS FRACTURE

WHAT IT IS: A stress fracture is a slight break in a bone brought on by repetitive stress. (In the military, they're known as march fractures.) With runners, the bones of the feet and lower legs are the most common sites for these. In the early stages, you might feel the sensation of a tugging ache. As the fracture worsens, pain will increase to the point it becomes more noticeable every time your affected leg lands.

Stress fractures are best confirmed by an MRI, but more severe ones can appear on an x-ray. It's worth pursuing that level of medical care if your bone pain is extremely sharp and centered on a small area (about the size of a dime or nickel).

SHORT-TERM TREATMENT: You can't finesse your way through a stress fracture. Continuing to run on one will just make it bigger. You'll need to stop

WHO TO SEE ABOUT RUNNING INJURIES

It can be tricky finding a good sports medicine professional to consult when you're injured. Word of mouth from fellow runners is often the best way to learn about physicians and others who will understand how important it is for you to get back to running, and then help you get there. If you can't get recommendations from others, look for specialists with a sports medicine certification in their field.

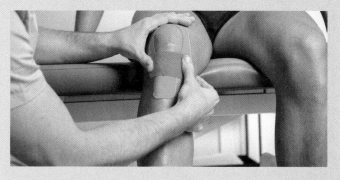

ORTHOPEDISTS AND OSTEO-PATHS: These are two of the main types of specialists runners see about injuries, especially when it's the knee. Orthopedists use imaging and in-person observations to diagnose acute injuries. If your injury is severe enough to merit surgery, the procedure is likely to be performed by an orthopedist.

Osteopaths are generally trained more holistically than orthopedists. If you have a recurrent injury that hasn't responded to conventional treatment, they might be able to unearth how an injury in one body part is related to a deficiency elsewhere.

PODIATRISTS: A good sports medicine podiatrist can do a lot more than treat your feet. If you have recurring knee and lower-leg injuries, that could well be because of a problem with your feet and ankles. Podiatrists can help you run with a sounder structure via better shoe selection, custom inserts, gait retraining, and foot and ankle exercise programs. Consider seeing a podiatrist for injuries such as Achilles tendinitis, plantar fasciitis, and foot and lower-leg stress fractures.

PHYSICAL THERAPISTS: Physical therapists can be a runner's best sports-med friend. They're not supposed to make medical diagnoses, but if you have a chronic low-level issue that detracts from your running, a physical therapist can often uncover it. They're trained to look at how the whole body moves, and to be alert to how an injury in one place stems from weakness or restriction elsewhere. A physical therapist will provide a targeted, progressive program to address the underlying problem.

CHIROPRACTORS: Some runners swear by chiropractors; others swear at them. Chiropractors can be a great help if your injury stems from problems in your pelvis or spine, especially structural issues such as one leg being shorter than the other. Beware, however, of chiropractors who want you to commit to several visits and tell you the only way to conquer your injury is to see them.

running for at least a few weeks, and possibly longer, depending on the site of the fracture, its severity, and how long you've been running on it.

You might need to avoid all weight-bearing on the injured leg for the early part of your recovery. That's more often the case for stress fractures of the feet than those elsewhere. You can usually find an alternative exercise that won't aggravate the injury, such as water running or others with little to no weight-bearing.

LONG-TERM PREVENTION: The two injury-avoidance principles noted—lessening the stress and strengthening the structure—are key to avoiding future stress fractures. Run on soft surfaces and wear shoes with adequate cushioning for your needs. Build your body's resistance by working on your running form and foot and lower-leg strength, and make sure you're getting adequate bone-health nutrients, especially calcium and vitamin D.

ACHILLES TENDINITIS

WHAT IT IS: As the name implies, this injury involves inflammation of the Achilles tendon, which attaches the calf muscles to the back of the heel. You'll feel tightness and/or pain in the tendon, especially after you've been stationary for a while and when running faster and uphill. You might also have visible swelling of the tendon and reddened skin in the area from the inflammation.

SHORT-TERM TREATMENT: In mild cases, you can keep doing short, slow runs, ideally on flat surfaces. You might find the tendon feels a little better after a bit of running. Stay under the amount of running that causes more discomfort in the area. Good calf stretching before running and several minutes of icing after are a must.

In more severe cases, you'll notice running will be immediately painful and/or compromised (in terms of being able to run with your normal gait).

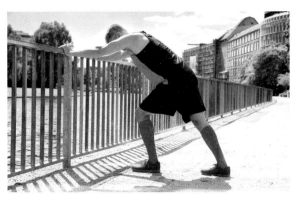

Calf stretch.

You'll need to stop running until short, easy jogs with your usual running form are pain-free.

LONG-TERM PREVENTION: Achilles tendinitis is common in runners with tight calf muscles. Make regular calf stretching (before and after every run) part of your routine. If you wear heeled shoes when not running, gradually transition to flatter shoes, so that your calves spend less time in a shortened position.

The other key to preventing a recurrence of this condition is strengthening the Achilles tendon. Do calf raises with a twist: place your hands on a table or countertop, rise up on your toes (of both feet), but lower yourself, slowly, only on the injured leg. Do twenty-five to fifty raises.

PLANTAR FASCIITIS

WHAT IT IS: The plantar fascia is a band of tissue that runs from the heel to the front of the foot. It can become inflamed and develop small tears when overworked. Plantar fascia usually starts as discomfort or pain in the bottom of the heel bone, especially on the inside. You might feel it most when you're barefoot and have been stationary for a while; pain upon getting out of bed is a classic symptom. You might not notice it running in the early stages of a race, but then the area will often be stiff and painful after your run.

THE PSYCHOLOGICAL SIDE OF INJURIES

Being an injured runner is trying. One of your main sources of joy, satisfaction, and stress relief is now another thing to worry about. And you will worry. Even if you've overcome previous injuries, you just know that, this time, things are different, and your days as a capable, carefree runner are over forever.

Relax. Take a deep breath. Yes, being injured stinks. But the odds are overwhelmingly in your favor that you'll be able to return to your normal running schedule soon. Some of what you should do as an injured runner is physical—the right rehabilitative exercises, a cautious return to running, and so on. Your psychological approach is also important. Having the right mindset will help you

on both a day-to-day and long-term basis when you're injured.

Look at your injury as a project and an opportunity. It's a project in that you can work toward the goal of "returning to normal running" as you would methodically attack any other challenge and goal. And it's an opportunity in that it's a chance to learn from your experience and figure out how to avoid being in this situation again.

Having that perspective will certainly help you better navigate your downtime than an understandable but unhelpful "this sucks" attitude. Every day will now have a purpose, as you progress toward healthy running. Think of each day's rehab work as a gift to yourself,

something that will hasten the return of doing what you want.

If your injury allows aerobic cross-training, try not to get overwhelmed by thoughts like, "What, I have to cycle indoors every day for the next three weeks?!" Find a way to get through each day's workout. One good trick is to imagine yourself going to bed that evening. Will you be happier with yourself if you worked out or blew it off? You can also lessen the monotony by varying your cross-training, with shorter and longer workouts, as well as stringing together easier and harder days of exercising during the recovery process.

Another way to help your psyche when you're injured? Try not to gain unwanted weight. Remind yourself that being at a better weight will make your return to running that much easier when that blessed time comes.

Finally, use this time to reflect on what you like most about running. It's often when something is denied us that we can best appreciate it. Vow never to complain about "having" to run again or otherwise take it for granted.

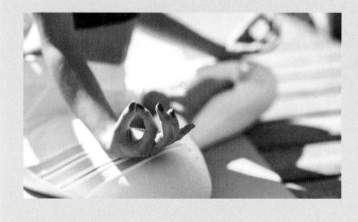

RUNNING AND MENSTRUATION

 Training quality and racing performance will be affected by the fluctuating hormones during your menstrual cycle, but you can work with it rather than feel limited by it.

The week leading up to your period is the high-hormone phase, so you may have a harder time regulating body temperature. Your electrolyte balance may also need more attention, and you may have achy body parts due to circulating prostaglandins (hormonelike substances that are involved in inflammation and other bodily processes).

These are things to address rather than ignore. You can make some changes via hydration strategies, targeted nutrition, and an anti-inflammatory so that you can still train or race well that week. In fact, exercise often reduces overly intense premenstrual symptoms.

During the week of your period you may feel rough. But keep in mind that you're in the low-hormone phase—and in that regard primed for a good race! World records such as Paula Radcliffe's former marathon mark of 2:15 have been set by people during the week of their periods, so don't let that keep you from getting out there.

Your menstrual cycle regularity is one of the barometers of your energy balance. If you notice a skipped cycle as your training is increasing, make sure you're getting enough specific macronutrients (especially protein and carbohydrates) and calories in your diet.

If you're approaching or past menopause, your changing hormone profile may be sabotaging your muscular gains. Increasing your dietary protein intake, especially the muscle-building branch chain amino acids, however, like leucine, can help you maintain muscular strength.

—*Molly Huddle,*
Olympian and American
record holder for 10,000
meters and the half marathon

SHORT-TERM TREATMENT: Short, slow runs are okay if your heel doesn't become more painful the longer you're out there. Long-term cases require rest until you can run without any pain in your heel. Stretch your calves and plantar fascia before and after running. Ice your heel after running as well. Throughout the day, massage-roll your heel with a self-massage tool or a lacrosse ball.

LONG-TERM PREVENTION: Plantar fasciitis is often caused by poor foot control when running. It's an example of an injury that happens to one body part because of weakness elsewhere. Improving your hip-flexor flexibility and strengthening your glutes and trunk will provide a more stable base for when your foot lands and pushes off during a run.

PIRIFORMIS SYNDROME (AND OTHER PAINS IN THE BUTT)

WHAT IT IS: Runners often complain about a combination of tightness, tugging, discomfort, point tenderness, and restriction in their hips and the sides of their glutes. This low-grade, sometimes chronic condition is often worse during periods of higher mileage. It's often especially bad during long periods of sitting.

Many people self-diagnose this discomfort as sciatica (impingement of the sciatic nerve by glute muscles) or piriformis syndrome (injury to the piriformis, one of the small glute muscles). But the same symptoms can arise when any of the glute muscles, especially the smaller ones, get overworked.

SHORT-TERM TREATMENT: You can usually keep running through this injury; in fact, many runners find that if they take time off, their problems return worse than ever when they resume training. While symptoms are especially bad, avoid long and hard runs, stretch before and after running, ice after running, and try to run on soft, flat surfaces. You can also get relief by gently rolling the affected area with a tennis or lacrosse ball. (It can be difficult to pinpoint the problem area with a larger device such as a foam roller.)

LONG-TERM PREVENTION: These problems almost always stem from weakness in the hips and glutes. That weakness leads to greater trunk instability when you run, with the small glute muscles taking on more work than they can handle. So, regular strengthening of those areas is key. Two other long-term measures to consider when battling this ailment are to improve your sitting posture and decrease the amount of time you spend sitting. Doing both will help prevent a tilted pelvis, which can make glute/hip weakness worse.

MUSCLE STRAIN

WHAT IT IS: Torn muscles of the sort you see in major-league sports—a sudden rupture of the muscle, leading to immobilization—are exceedingly rare in distance running. We tend to get micro-tears that develop over time. These slight tears are usually felt as a strain or tugging sensation in the muscle; you'll feel restricted, unable to move through a full range of motion. The most

common sites for these are the calves, quadriceps, and where the hamstrings connect to the pelvis.

SHORT-TERM TREATMENT: It's okay to keep running if your muscle strain doesn't alter your running form. Stick to short, easy runs on flat surfaces. Ice affected areas after you run and a couple other times during the day. And this is really important: Don't stretch the affected area! This isn't a case of your muscle being tight, in which case stretching will help. While the muscle is in an acute strained phase, stretching it, especially before you run, will just aggravate it.

LONG-TERM PREVENTION: These strains usually develop because of muscular weakness. Consult a physical therapist or a licensed athletic trainer about a targeted strengthening program for the muscle and its surrounding area.

This and the preceding chapters have shown you how to be a healthy, happy, capable runner. Now let's turn to enjoying your running even more, the runDisney way.

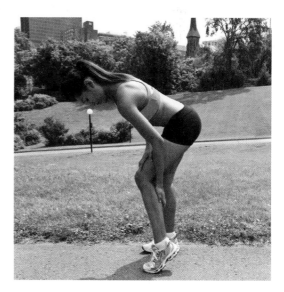

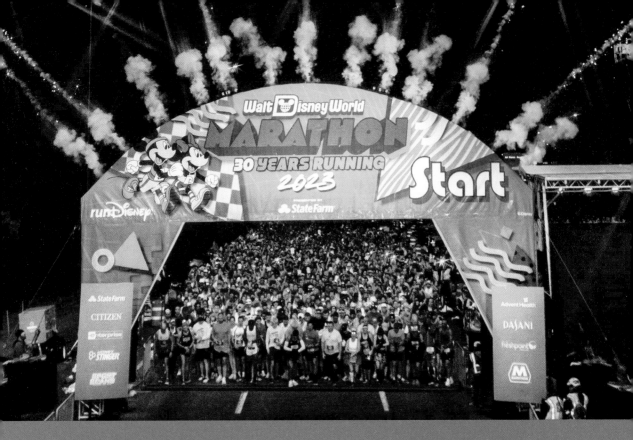

CHAPTER 6:
THE RUNDOWN ON RUNDISNEY EVENTS

A runDisney race is anything but ordinary.

How does this sound? Start with fireworks bursting overhead. Run through Disney theme parks that are lined with Disney characters and have live entertainment going on simultaneously. Share the road with fellow Disney enthusiasts clad in costumes. Ultimately, crossing the finish line and being rewarded with a commemorative medal inspired by the runDisney weekend theme. And, if you want, do it all again the following day, when you take part in the multirace challenge offered at each runDisney event. (We'll look at how to prepare for these unique events in chapter 9.)

In this chapter, we'll look at all runDisney events, in the order in which they're held each year, followed by how to plan your Disney "runcation." For more information, and to register, see rundisney.com/events. We hope to see you there!

HOW IT ALL GOT STARTED

Disney is synonymous with imagination. That's as true in the running arena as it is in movies and other endeavors.

The first runDisney races were held in 1994, after years of behind-the-scenes planning to produce a world-class event. The inaugural weekend run event consisted of the Walt Disney World Marathon, plus a two-mile fun run for those wanting to run a shorter distance. Race organizers realized runDisney could offer something that even marquee events couldn't match—a running tour of the world's most famous theme parks. Just how brilliant was the idea? Well, Fred Lebow, the visionary behind the five-borough New York City Marathon, loved the concept the moment he heard it, and served as honorary race chair that first year.

At a time when marathons and most other road races were still focused primarily on the fast folks up front, runDisney took a different approach. The inaugural Walt Disney World Marathon was the first large marathon to feature world-class entertainment throughout the course. The emphasis on fun and everyday runners was a major contributor to what became known as the second running boom. (The first running boom, triggered by events such as American Frank Shorter's Olympic Marathon win at the 1972 Munich games, started in the early 1970s, and was more focused on competitive running.) Participation in organized races skyrocketed during the 1990s and early 2000s as many events followed runDisney's lead.

The Walt Disney World Half Marathon was added in 1998 to meet the rising demand for a runDisney event that didn't cover 26.2 miles. Initially, the half marathon and marathon were run on the same day, plus started at the same time. Marathoners finished at EPCOT, while those in the half marathon concluded their run at the Magic Kingdom. An Family Fun 5K was also added for Thursday.

But then a funny thing happened: Runners in both races were having such a great time that they didn't want to have to choose between the half marathon and marathon. They wanted to do both. So, the half marathon was moved to the day before the marathon. Race organizers expected a few hundred people at most to take on the challenge of a 13.1-mile run on Saturday and a 26.2-mile run on Sunday. Instead, more than 2,500 signed up to do just that almost immediately!

Thus was born the Goofy Challenge. Still, some runners wanted additional opportunities to run through Walt Disney World. More races on more days were added, and eventually the Dopey Challenge—a 5K on Thursday, a 10K on Friday, then a half marathon on Saturday, and a marathon on Sunday—became an official happening. These challenges became such an integral part of the runDisney experience that races throughout the year feature them.

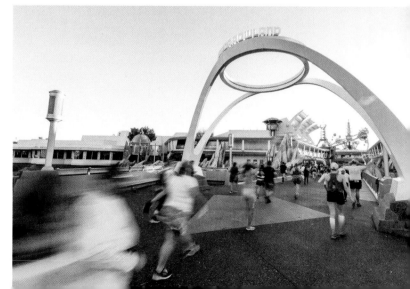

WALT DISNEY WORLD MARATHON WEEKEND

WHEN: Early January
WHERE: Walt Disney World Resort, Florida

This is the one that started it all! The Walt Disney World Marathon was first run in 1994, with the half marathon, now run on the preceding day, added in 1998. The weekend celebrates all things Disney—and with four races in four days, there's plenty of time to celebrate. The Walt Disney World Marathon is the longest race in the runDisney portfolio. The weekend also features the longest challenge distance of the runDisney race season. The early January date means you'll be doing the bulk of your training during the fall, when most feel perfect running weather prevails.

STAND-ALONE RACE OVERVIEW

THURSDAY, 5:00 A.M.: Walt Disney World 5K
Usual field size: 14,000

FRIDAY, 5:00 A.M.: Walt Disney World 10K
Usual field size: 14,000

SATURDAY, 5:00 A.M.: Walt Disney World Half Marathon
Usual field size: 22,000

SUNDAY, 5:00 A.M.: Walt Disney World Marathon
Usual field size: 15,000

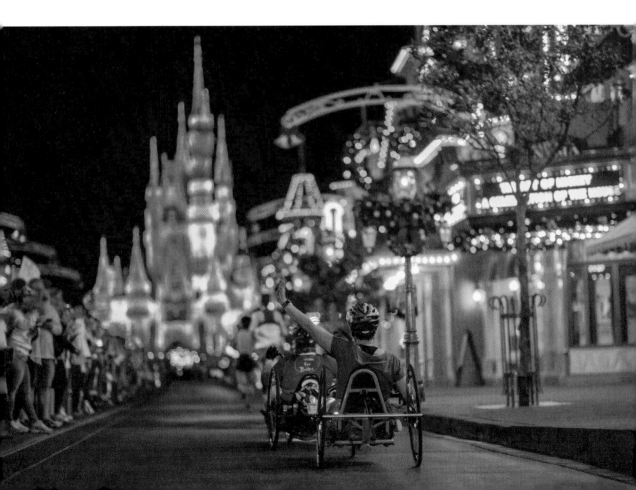

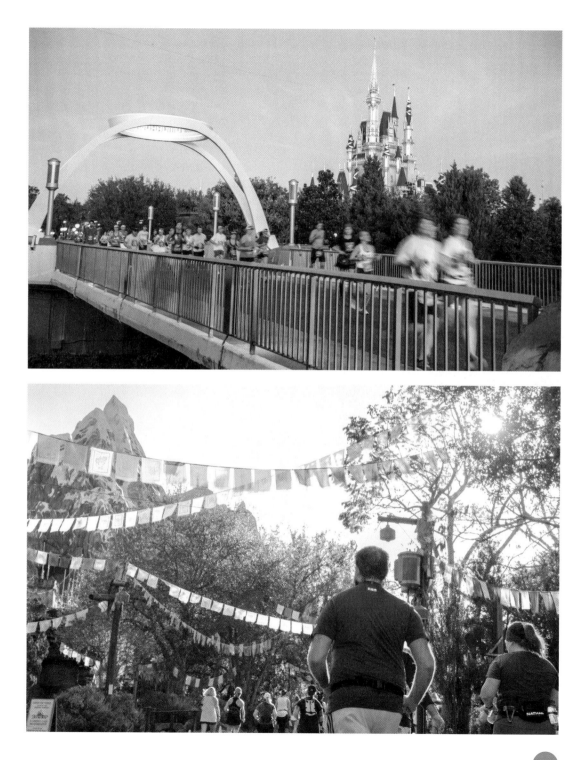

PACE YOURSELF

For all runDisney races, participants must maintain a 16:00 minute per mile pace or faster to earn a finisher's medal. Here's what that pace works out to for finishing times in the race distances offered:

- 5K: 49:42
- 10K: 1:39:25
- 10-miler: 2:40
- Half Marathon: 3:29:45
- Marathon: 6:59:30

WEEKEND CHALLENGE

Make that two challenges! Goofy's Race and a Half Challenge calls on participants to run the half marathon on Saturday and the marathon on Sunday—a total of 39.3 miles. Those brave enough to take on the Dopey Challenge and run each race offered garner a total of 48.6 miles over four days.

Goofy's Race and a Half Challenge was first run in 2006, and proved to be so popular that all runDisney weekends now include a multi-race challenge. Runners who complete both races on pace earn a Goofy's Race and a Half Challenge medal in addition to the half marathon and marathon medals. You'll need to register for Goofy's Race and a Half Challenge to be eligible for the challenge medal. More than 7,500 runners now usually tackle this endeavor.

The Dopey Challenge was added in 2014 to accommodate runners who want it all. To reiterate, you'll do the 5K on Thursday, the 10K on Friday, a half marathon on Saturday, and the marathon on Sunday. Complete the challenge, and you'll go home with six finisher medals: one from each individual race, one for the Goofy's Race and a Half Challenge, and one for the Dopey Challenge.

You'll need to register for the Dopey Challenge to be eligible for the specific Dopey Challenge medal. The field for this multi-race pursuit usually totals more than six thousand hearty souls!

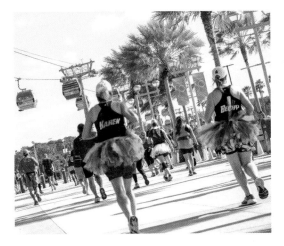

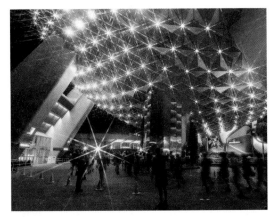

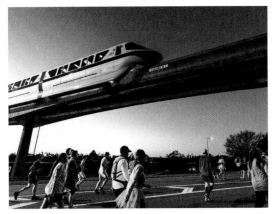

CELEBRATE FAMILY FITNESS WITH KIDS RACES

Some runDisney events at the Disneyland Resort in California include a full slate of kids races as well. In all, about three thousand young runners usually take part.

The kids races, held late morning and early afternoon on the Saturday of race week end, are open to children nine and younger. (Parents can also participate.) All kids get a finisher medallion and receive lots of support from their favorite Disney characters.

The ages and distances for participants break down in the following categories:

- 12 months and under: Diaper Dash
- 1–4 years old: 100-meter dash
- 5–8 years old: 200-meter dash

Following these dashes is the runDisney Kids One Mile Run.

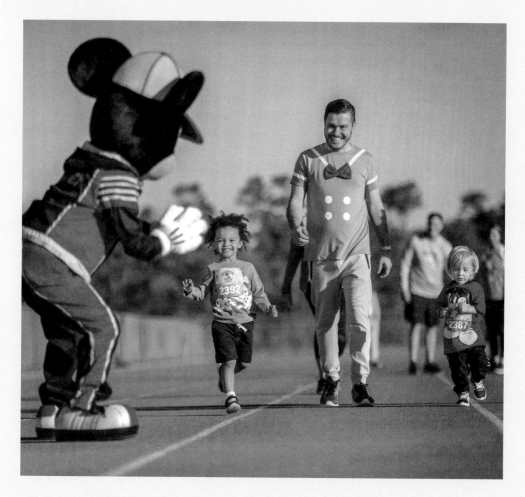

DISNEYLAND HALF MARATHON WEEKEND

WHEN: January
WHERE: Disneyland Resort, California

The runDisney magic returns to the Disneyland Resort for a January weekend of events including a 5K, 10K, and half marathon through Disneyland Park and Disney California Adventure Park. The packed weekend also includes an early-morning yoga session, races for kids, and the Dumbo Double Dare Challenge.

STAND-ALONE RACE OVERVIEW

FRIDAY: Disneyland 5K

SATURDAY: Disneyland 10K

SUNDAY: Disneyland Half Marathon

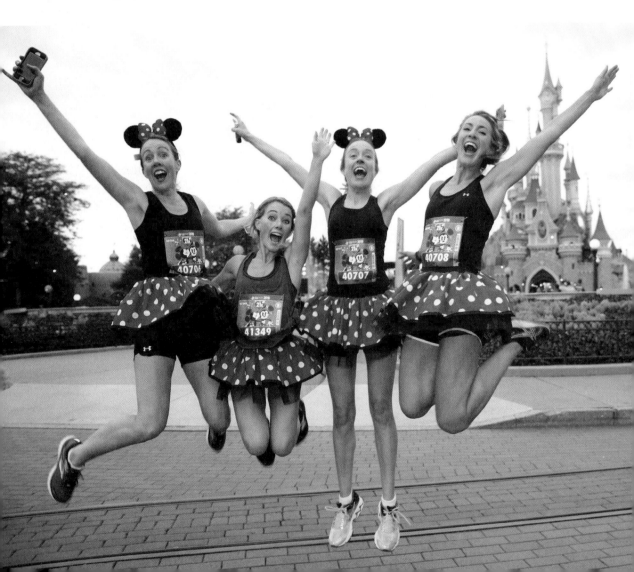

TAKE ON A COAST-TO-COAST CHALLENGE!

Beginning in 2024, runners who complete any 10-mile race—or longer—at both Walt Disney World Resort and the Disneyland Resort in the same calendar year will receive a runDisney Coast to Coast Race Challenge medal.

Guests will not need to register for the runDisney Coast to Coast Race Challenge as a separate registration.

- Both qualifying races must be completed in the same calendar year.
- Guests only earn one runDisney Coast to Coast Race Challenge medal per calendar year.
- runDisney Coast to Coast Race Challenge medals will be available after crossing the finish line of the second race.
- Guests must be fourteen years or older to participate.
- Participation in virtual races does not count toward eligibility for the runDisney Coast to Coast Race Challenge medal.

DUMBO DOUBLE DARE CHALLENGE

The Dumbo Double Dare Challenge combines Saturday's Disneyland 10K with Sunday's Disneyland Half Marathon for a total of 19.3 miles.

Runners who complete each course within the allotted time earn the finisher medals for each individual race as well as a special Dumbo Double Dare Challenge medal.

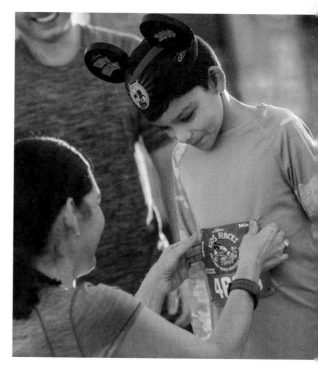

KIDS RACES

Every child nine or younger who participates in the Kids Races goes home a winner with a finisher medallion designed for the tiniest of runners. There's even a Diaper Dash for crawlers.

runDisney Kids Races are open to children up to age nine. Kids Races will be broken down into the following age groups:

- 🐭 Ages 0–1
- 🐭 Ages 1–3
- 🐭 Ages 4–6
- 🐭 Ages 7–9

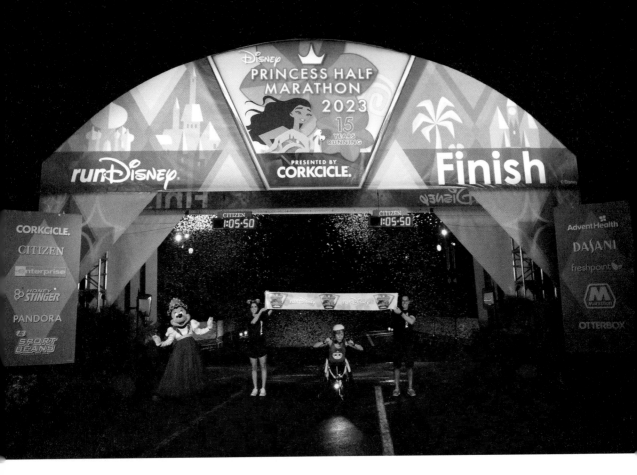

DISNEY PRINCESS HALF MARATHON WEEKEND

WHEN: Late February
WHERE: Walt Disney World Resort, Florida

Since 2009, the Disney Princess Half Marathon Weekend has put a Disney spin on celebrating women's running. There's certainly no mistaking the princess theme—you'll never see more runners in tutus than what you'll come across at this weekend event. Princess Weekend has become known among runners as *the* weekend-with-friends destination event. Don't let the name fool you—princes are welcome, too. The late February date makes this event a great excuse to escape winter for a weekend in Florida.

STAND-ALONE RACE OVERVIEW

FRIDAY, 5:00 A.M.: Disney Princess 5K
Usual field size: 13,500

SATURDAY, 5:00 A.M.: Disney Princess 10K
Usual field size: 14,500

SUNDAY, 5:00 A.M.: Disney Princess Half Marathon
Usual field size: 25,000

ON-COURSE OFFERINGS

Proper hydration and fueling help you run your best. All runDisney events at the Walt Disney World Resort and Disneyland Resort include water stops. The longer races feature more stops and also offer sports drinks, food, and medical tents.

The Disney Princess 5K, 10K, and Half Marathon are run on essentially the same courses as the Walt Disney World 5K, 10K, and Half Marathon.

But while the courses are the same, the on-course experiences aren't. The runDisney entertainment team themes the races completely differently for Disney Princess Weekend. The result: all the great landmarks of the January races, but with a unique theme.

WEEKEND CHALLENGE

The Disney Fairytale Challenge (originally called the Glass Slipper Challenge) was added in 2014 for those who *really* want to test their endurance and attain racing royalty status. Run the Disney Princess 10K on Saturday and the Disney Princess Half Marathon on Sunday for a total of 19.3 miles. Completing both races on pace gets you the Disney Fairytale Challenge medal in addition to the 10K and Half Marathon finisher medals.

You'll need to register for the Disney Fairytale Challenge, which includes both races, for your runs to be recognized and for you to earn the Fairytale Challenge medal. There are usually more than 8,500 Disney Fairytale Challenge runners.

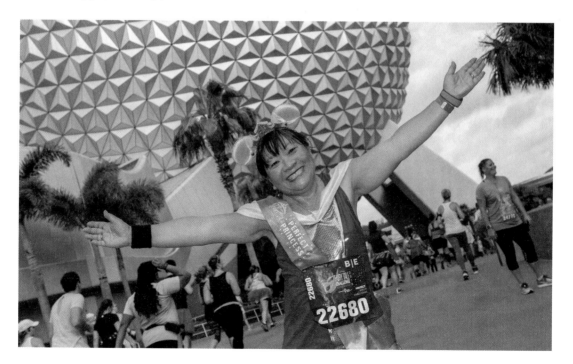

RUNDISNEY RACE ETIQUETTE

 The freedom of running is wonderful, and the festive atmosphere at runDisney events is exciting. But as in all large-crowd situations, there are certain rules of the road that everyone needs to follow to maintain efficient traffic flow and reduce collisions and bottlenecks.

When taking a walk break, gently move over to the right side, while being aware of other runners around you.

Signal to fellow runners that you're taking a walk break. It helps to have a timer that has a loud beep. Set this for a five-beep countdown. When the countdown starts, wave your hand as you move over to the side of the road to walk. Once you do this a few times your fellow runners will understand.

When congregating at water stations, move to one side or the other to take water or walk. Leave the center of the road open for those who are running through.

When stopping at a toilet or for a Disney character photo, look ahead, behind, left, and right, and ease your way over to the side of the road.

When returning to the race after a stop, look at the runners behind approaching who are running by, find an opening, and ease back into the stream.

When running with a friend or a group, run single file in narrow areas. Even when there's more room on the road, groups should be courteous to other runners

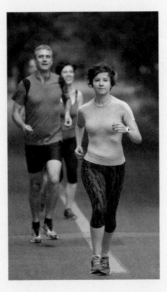

by running no more than two abreast.

When getting rid of clothing, costumes, etc., move gradually to the side of the road and toss your objects clear of the road or edge, where runners might be running. As described elsewhere in this chapter, these clothes will be collected and donated to local charities.

If you plan to wear a costume, look at the runDisney rules. Realize that you'll be in crowded conditions where projections like Tinker Bell's wings might be in someone's face.

Avoid wearing any garment that has string, ropes, or clothing that would drag along the ground.

—*Jeff Galloway,*
Olympian and official
runDisney training consultant

RUNDISNEY SPRINGTIME SURPRISE WEEKEND

WHEN: Mid-April
WHERE: Walt Disney World Resort, Florida

A different theme, hence the word "surprise" in the name of the event, awaits runners each year in this new annual entry on the runDisney calendar. An early-morning yoga session kicks off the weekend's events. The mid-April date provides just the incentive you need to hit spring running.

STAND-ALONE RACE OVERVIEW

FRIDAY, 5:00 A.M.: runDisney Springtime Surprise 5K
Usual field size: 13,500

SATURDAY, 5:00 A.M.: runDisney Springtime Surprise 10K
Usual field size: 13,000

SUNDAY, 5:00 A.M.: runDisney Springtime Surprise 10-Miler
Usual field size: 14,000

WEEKEND CHALLENGE

The runDisney Springtime Surprise Challenge combines the Springtime Surprise 5K on Friday, the Springtime Surprise 10K on Saturday, and the Springtime Surprise 10-Miler on Sunday for a combined total of 19.3 miles.

Runners must register for the Springtime Surprise Challenge to earn the challenge medal (which comes along with their finisher medals from the 5K, 10K, and 10-Miler).

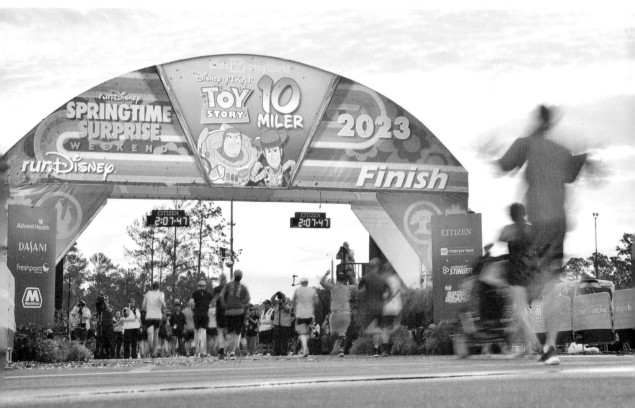

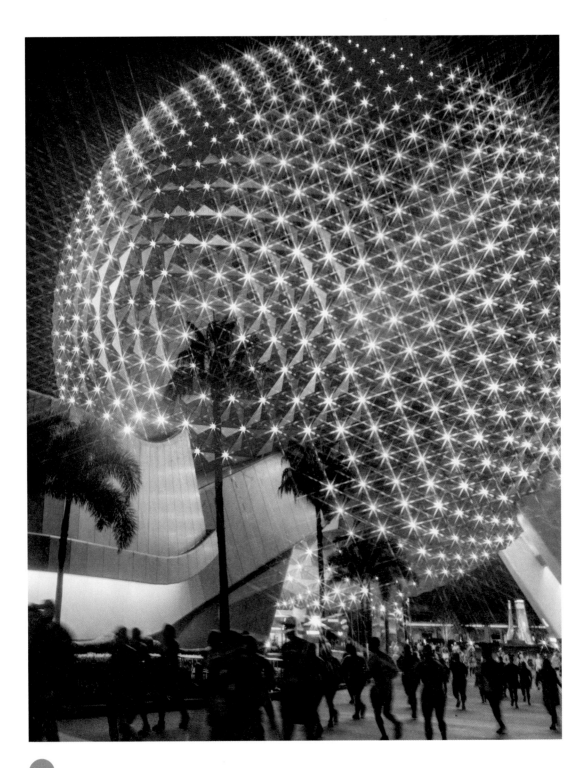

TOP FIVE MISTAKES IN RACE-DAY PACING

My run-walk-run method has helped thousands enjoy— and finish!—runDisney races. One reason these runners have a great time is that they properly pace themselves. To get the most out of your runDisney experience, avoid these common pacing mistakes.

STARTING TOO FAST: Use the first mile or two to warm up. Go slower and walk more during this period to let the legs, feet, etc., acclimate to the increased exertion level of running you'll be establishing. Logistics can help you with this tip: the first mile of all large events is very crowded, so let the congestion ease up before you really get your legs moving.

NOT TAKING WALK BREAKS FROM THE BEGINNING: Adjusting to a conservative run-walk-run strategy from the start can help keep postponing fatigue for many miles. If you run three miles before taking a walk break, you won't erase those three miles of fatigue. This often results in a slowdown during the last few miles.

RUNNING TOO FAST AFTER A STOP: It's common to want to make up time after a bathroom break or a photo op with a runDisney character. Doing so is especially tempting if you're running with a friend who doesn't stop. The better approach is to go with the flow of the runners around you and enjoy the entertainment and the energy of other runners. Take a mile or more to gradually catch up.

BEING TOO FOCUSED ON PACE: If you're looking only at your watch, you'll miss a lot of the fun. Enjoy each display and character. A high percentage of your fellow runners will be wearing costumes and adding to the festive moments. (It's only if you're concerned about

finishing the course in the allotted time that you should monitor pace at each mile to stay ahead of the back-of-the-pack balloon runner ladies [who are just in front of the pickup vans].)

NOT HAVING A PACING PLAN: During the week before your race, look at your "magic mile" pace predictions and select a conservative plan for each mile. Saving resources by pacing and employing a run-walk-run plan from the beginning is smart and probably affords you the opportunity to pass a lot of spent runners during the last few miles.

—Jeff Galloway,
Olympian and official
runDisney training consultant

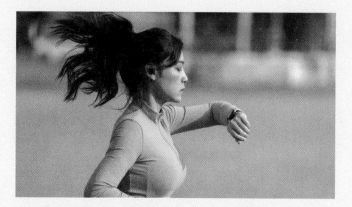

DISNEY WINE & DINE HALF MARATHON WEEKEND

WHEN: First weekend of November
WHERE: Walt Disney World Resort, Florida

Foodies will enjoy the half marathon, which was first run in 2010. Any (or all!) of the races are a great way to work up an appetite for a celebration of the fall harvest. The early November date is the perfect focus before the busy holiday season gets underway.

STAND-ALONE RACE OVERVIEW

FRIDAY, 5:00 A.M.: Disney Wine & Dine 5K
Usual field size: 5,000

SATURDAY, 5:00 A.M.: Disney Wine & Dine 10K
Usual field size: 12,500

SUNDAY, 5:00 A.M.: Wine & Dine Half Marathon
Usual field size: 16,000

WEEKEND CHALLENGE

First run in 2016, the Disney Two Course Challenge combines the 10K on Saturday with the half marathon on Sunday for a total of 19.3 miles. Runners who complete both races on pace earn the Disney Two Course Challenge medal in addition to the 10K and half marathon medals.

Runners must register for the Disney Two Course Challenge to be eligible for the challenge medal. About 6,500 runners typically take on this challenge.

The Post-Race Party allows runners a chance to celebrate and enjoy the EPCOT International Food & Wine Festival. Half Marathon and Challenge registration includes entry. Friends and family can purchase Post-Race Party tickets to attend the private event.

VIRTUAL SUMMER SERIES

Virtual races are a great introduction to the magic of runDisney. Just like in the races at the Walt Disney World Resort and Disneyland Resort, you wear a bib and get a commemorative medal when you finish. The twist is that you pick the course—around your neighborhood, in a local park, or at the nearest track. Then you submit your results, print your finisher's certificate, and get your medal.

There are two distinct virtual race offerings.

Over the summer, there's the runDisney Virtual Series—5K races (3.1 miles) available in June, July, and August. These races are perfect for beginning runners or anyone who wants to set a goal to work toward. Each race has a unique Disney theme, and a special finisher's medal to match. You can also do a summer-long challenge: finish all three virtual 5Ks, and you'll get a separate medal for your achievement.

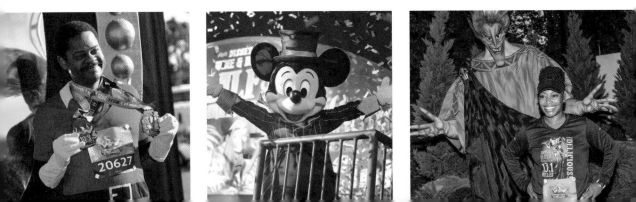

RUNNING RUNDISNEY TO HELP OTHERS

Make the world a little better while having the experience of a lifetime? What's not to like?

You can partner with one of more than twenty participating charities to gain entry to a runDisney event. To do so, you agree to raise a minimum amount of money to help fund the charity's work. The select group of charities includes organizations that fund disease research and provide education and awareness on both childhood and adult diseases. For a full list, see rundisney.com.

Separately, runDisney and runners raise hundreds of thousands of dollars each year to support local and national charities, including Second Harvest Food Bank of Central Florida, the Leukemia & Lymphoma Society, and Make-A-Wish Central and Northern Florida.

Oh, and the clothes you might wear to the start and discard once you're running? They'll be collected and put to good use; thousands of pounds of clothing gathered at runDisney races have been donated to charity.

RUNDISNEY VIRTUAL 12KS OF CHRISTMAS

Deck your running shoes for this holiday-themed challenge. The 12Ks of Christmas includes three 4K races (and a Challenge) providing a perfect opportunity for families and friends to get together for a little holiday Disney magic—wherever they run. And each medal doubles as a Christmas ornament. In addition to customizable digital tools such as themed race bibs and finisher certificates, racers in this series also receive new and exclusive offerings like a long-sleeve shirt, and a Corkcicle mug and hot cocoa kit for those chilly winter nights.

- Participants must run three 4Ks to complete the Challenge.

- Participants need to complete all 4Ks between December 1 and December 31.

- The three 4Ks can be completed at any time and pace that is convenient to participants

AMENITIES

Participants who register for runDisney Virtual 12Ks of Christmas Challenge will receive:

- 4 ornaments as medals
- Long-sleeve shirt
- Chocolate Bomb
- Corkcicle mug
- Digital race bib
- Finisher certificates
- Digital tool kit

For more information on virtual races, see rundisney.com/events/virtual.

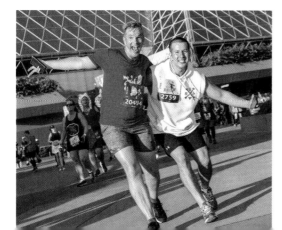

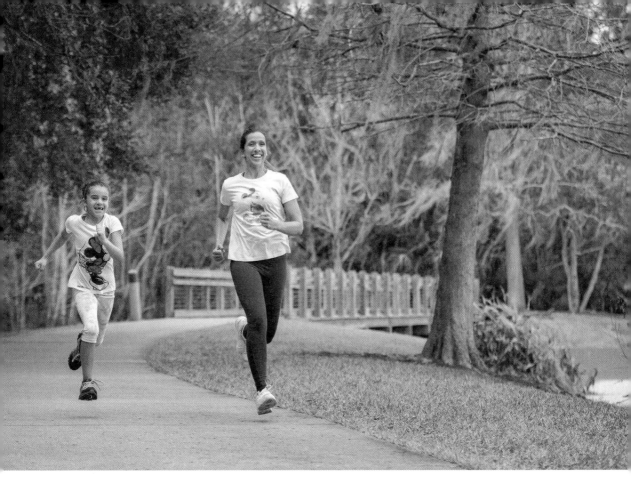

PLANNING YOUR RUNDISNEY RUNCATION

The best way to make your runDisney weekend truly magical? Plan to stay at the Walt Disney World Resort or Disneyland Resort for their events. You and your family will have a world of fun—and convenience—at your fingertips.

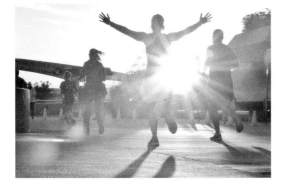

At Walt Disney World, there are more than twenty-five hotels to choose from (see the appendix in the back of the book) within the resort's grounds, each with its own theme and personality. On race weekend, they all have one important thing in common: they provide free shuttles to and from all race events.

Insider tip: At this time, all events at Walt Disney World start and finish at EPCOT. However, courses are subject to change. If you want to be showered and ready to tour the rest of the resort as soon as possible postrace, go with lodging in the EPCOT Resort Area.

Staying in the resort also gives you easy access to four theme parks: Magic Kingdom Park, EPCOT, Disney's Hollywood Studios, and Disney's Animal Kingdom Theme Park. Each park contains old

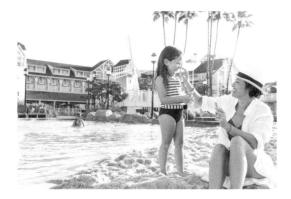

favorites and new and exciting lands like Toy Story Land and *Star Wars*: Galaxy's Edge.

You probably have your favorite pre- and post-race foods. And it's a safe bet you can find your favs at the more than four hundred restaurants located throughout the resort. Disney Dining options range from themed eateries, family buffets, and food trucks to dinner shows, tap houses, and bakeries, as well as anything else you could possibly have a craving for. If you run low on fuel

near the end of your race, it won't be for lack of carbo-loading opportunities available to you. (See the Appendix for a listing of where to find some of the healthier eating options at Walt Disney World and Disneyland Resort.)

Want to stretch your legs a little postrace, but not too much? Take one of the free shuttles to Disney Springs, a premier dining, shopping, and entertainment center. Four distinct neighborhoods make up the center, which is built around bubbling springs. Among the more than 150 offerings is the World of Disney store, which is the largest Disney character store in the world.

All of these race weekend options and opportunities are available by booking your resort stay through the Walt Disney Travel Company. When you plan your trip that way, you'll get extras such as theme park tickets, miniature golf vouchers, and discounts on dining and entertainment. (Park passes don't come with your runDisney race registration.)

Go to waltdisneyworld.com or disneyland.com

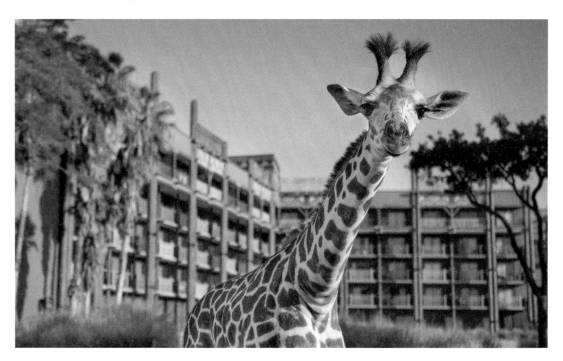

to find several planning tools, including MagicBands, which make park and room entrances super easy and Memory Maker, which gives you unlimited PhotoPass digital downloads of your weekend, including, of course, your runDisney event photos.

Of course, there are also several appealing off-resort lodging options within reasonable distance of the resort. (See the Appendix for a list of what we call Walt Disney World "good neighbor" hotels.)

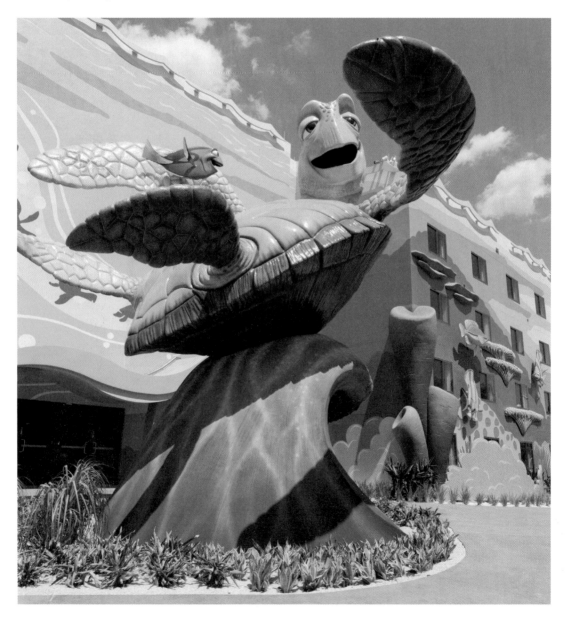

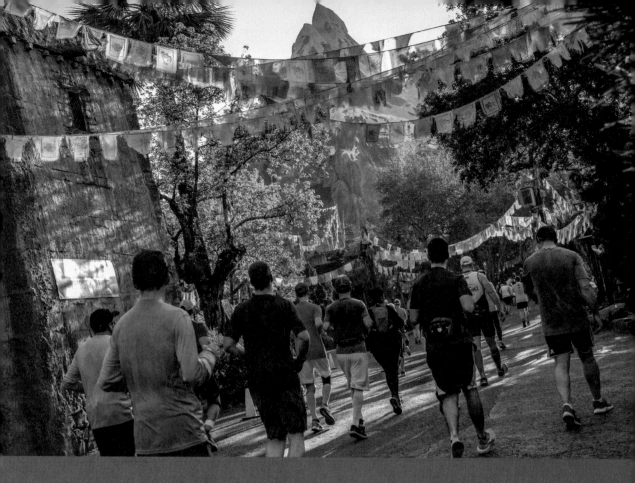

CHAPTER 7:
FIND YOUR
RUNDISNEY GROUP

A run by yourself is a great time to think things through, blow off steam, or simply zone out. We all need some good "me" time now and then.

Most of us also need good companionship, even when running. Finding a kindred spirit (or spirits) will improve your running—and life—immeasurably. You'll seldom have a better social hour than when running with friends and family, talking about everything and nothing while sharing effort and exerting yourself. Creating bonds with your fellow runners will give you support when you need it . . . and a cheering section when it's time to crow. You'll probably wind up with some of the deepest, most meaningful relationships of your life when engaged in a run.

Here's how to find your running group.

ISO RUNNING FRIENDS

How do you go about acquiring running partners? After all, it's unlikely you'll approach a stranger and say, "Tomorrow morning at five I'll be outside my house in not much clothing. Wanna swing by and sweat with me?"

Most running friendships develop organically. Runners know from personal experience we all need someone to lean on at times. Once you've made someone's acquaintance, it's well within common running etiquette to toss out the idea of getting together for a run. The other person is probably just as eager as you to have lots of people to run with.

If you have a somewhat set running schedule, you probably see a lot of the same people out running over and over. You might exchange waves, then greetings, then maybe a few words when passing one another. Eventually, one might ask the other, "Mind if I tag along for a few minutes?" Soon, you're making plans to run together. Many running friendships have sprung from these repeated encounters.

If you have one running partner, it's likely you probably have more potential running partners than you might think. Almost every runner knows other runners. Tap into those networks to

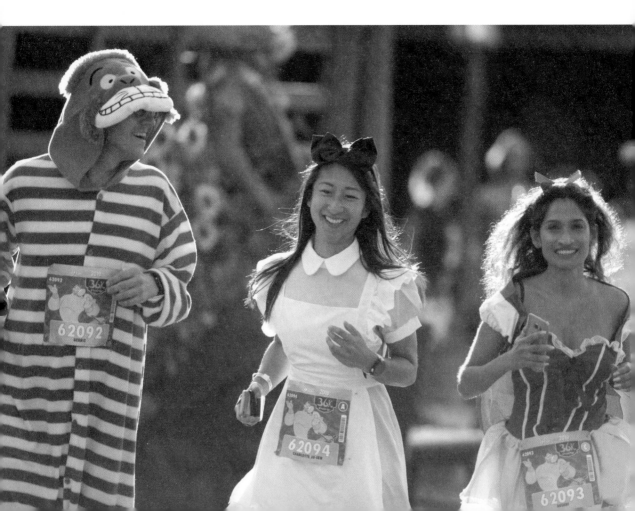

WHY AND HOW TO FIND TRAINING PARTNERS

 For synergy, fun, and added accountability, try doing at least some of your training with others.

Meeting a group or training partner for a run can make getting out the door easier (especially when there's bad weather or it's early in the morning).

The key is to find someone with similar goals to yours, so the pace, daily mileage, and overall training mesh well enough. If you don't match up exactly with your partner on pace or distance, try to work together on pieces of the run or workout. For example, you can do multiple loops and join your partner for either the first or second half if the person is going longer. If he or she is faster, maybe their "easy" day is your hard workout day, or vice versa. Running on the track is a great way to easily hop in and out of each other's workouts at different distances as well.

It's totally fine to sometimes want to do your easy-run days alone—to be mindful of your recovery efforts, to be alone with your thoughts, and to just flow at your own pace. However, as a whole, I find meeting up with someone when you can is more constructive, gets one more race-ready.

Group runs defuse the tension that can accompany harder or longer runs; you have someone to share stories, jokes, and encouraging words with. Plus, a windy day is only half as windy when you take turns in the lead and literally reduce drag as you drag each other to fitness. So, sign your friend, family member, or partner up for the race, too, and add some accountability, social enjoyment, support, and teamwork to your preparations!

—Molly Huddle,
Olympian and American
record holder for 10,000
meters and the half marathon

see if the schedules and typical runs of others align with yours. Being part of a group doing a long run is a great way to meet friends (and their friends). See if you click and make a connection.

A few other sources of potential training partners are these:

WORK: There will most likely be other runners at your job if you work in a large enough place. See if there's a group that heads out at lunch or at the end of the day. If not, start one.

LOCAL RUNNING CLUBS AND STORES: Most clubs and stores organize group runs. You'll naturally gravitate toward others around your pace. Commit to a few of these outings and see if you hit it off with anyone.

RACES: If you do a lot of local races, you'll eventually realize you keep finishing around the same people. These are great potential running partners because you already know you're roughly matched on pace with them. If you're comfortable doing so, introduce yourself, maybe invite the other person to join you for a cooldown jog, and see if running together might work.

And who knows . . . through one or more of these friends and connections, you just might find a few new runDisney fans to travel with to your next race event.

FIND FELLOW RUNDISNEY FANS

You're not just a runner, of course. You're a runDisney runner! Fortunately, it's easy to connect with your fellow aerobic Disney fans.

The runDisney social channels are a must here. Find your group on runDisney's Facebook, Twitter, Instagram, Pinterest, and YouTube accounts. For starters, you'll have the inside track on everything runDisney—event updates, weekend theme announcements, and more.

You'll also find inspiration and ideas for every aspect of your running. If you need a boost or want to boast, your fellow runners will be there for you. Holding yourself accountable to others online can be a great way to get through a rough run. Seeing others nail their training and reach their runDisney goals will motivate you to do the same. And if you come up short on costume ideas, you'll know where to turn.

You can further your runDisney connections with others by running for charity. See chapter 6 for more on that topic.

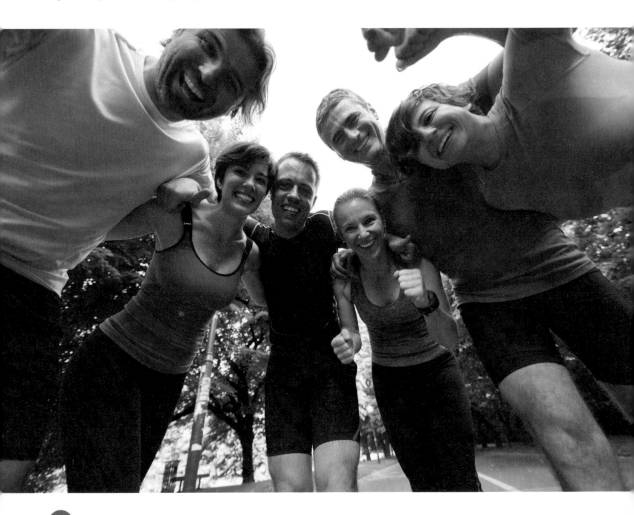

RUNNING WITH YOUR FOUR-LEGGED FRIEND

Dogs can be one of the best running partners you'll ever have. They're happy to go whatever time is best for you, and they'll never text you, "Sorry, need to cancel for the morning. Up late working."

Most breeds can handle some amount of regular running. Hunting dogs, working dogs, Labs, retrievers, and mutts who obviously have some of those genes are especially good. They're wired for activity.

No matter how active your dog has been, ease him into your running routine. The way we run is a little foreign to most dogs, who more typically sprint and trot and stop and smell than maintain a steady pace over a straightforward route. Start with one run together a week for a few weeks. If your dog seems to get the gist of what you're doing and to enjoy it, add another day together per week. On the days your dog doesn't run with you, let him set the tone for your outings.

Keep runs with your dog on the shorter side. Dogs don't sweat, and aren't as efficient as humans at dissipating heat. On his own,

your dog would slow or stop (and jump in water, if possible) if he started to overheat. Yes, he might be able to go for hours. But you don't want to find out after it's too late that he overdid it trying to keep up with you. Pay special attention to overheating if your dog has a thick coat.

If you want to run more than your dog on a given day, you can start with a couple miles together, then drop him off and carry on. Alternatively, do most of your run alone, then swing by the house and get your dog, and share the last few miles of your run with him.

Running with dogs is hardly a novelty; it's enough of a thing that there are leashes made for that purpose. Experiment to see what setup works for you and your pooch. What works best depends on many factors. Are you okay running with one end of the leash cinched around your waist, or do you feel you can run at a more normal gait holding one end of the leash? Does your dog dutifully trot alongside, or tend to pull? Will you be running where it's easy to navigate around obstacles

without getting tangled or running into danger?

In an ideal world—for you and your dog—you have access to places where the dog can run off-leash. You'll probably never see your dog happier than on these runs. Be sure he's listening to you at all times.

And while we're speaking of voice control—run with your dog at a conversational pace. You want to be able to communicate effectively with him at all times.

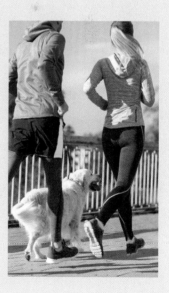

MAKE FITNESS A FAMILY AFFAIR

"Disney" and "family-friendly" are nearly synonymous. So, it makes perfect sense that "runDisney" and "family fitness" should also be inextricably linked.

Running can be a family affair regardless of everyone's ages. You might think you know everything there is to know about your partner, but you'll probably learn a few new things when you run together. Many couples cherish these times together as a unique way to bond. Others, it must be said, would use a word other than "cherish" to describe their joint workouts. Pro tip: for the good of the relationship, let the slower member of the couple set the pace.

Modern running strollers have allowed countless parents to keep up their running despite the demands of child care. If two parents can make the run, all the better, because you can take turns pushing. Some runners don't mind how pushing a stroller affects their form, while others will welcome the chance to use their arms normally. Remember that the little ones being pushed won't build up heat like you will; dress them accordingly. Sun protection for the tykes is a must.

Ignore people who might say you're being a bad parent (and an obsessive runner) by using a running stroller. Bringing your young children with you sends the message from an early age that being fit and active is a normal part of life.

When your children have the motor coordination to run at least a few hundred yards, what should you do? How can you best share your love for running with them?

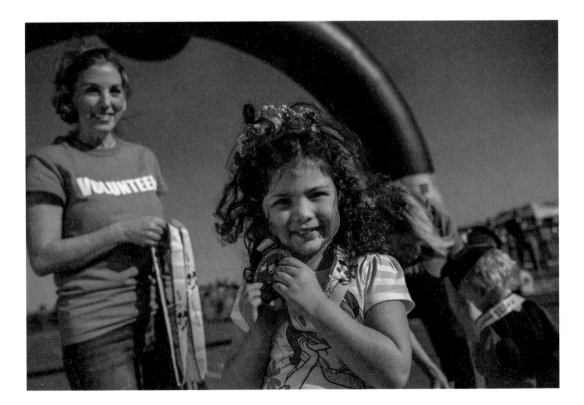

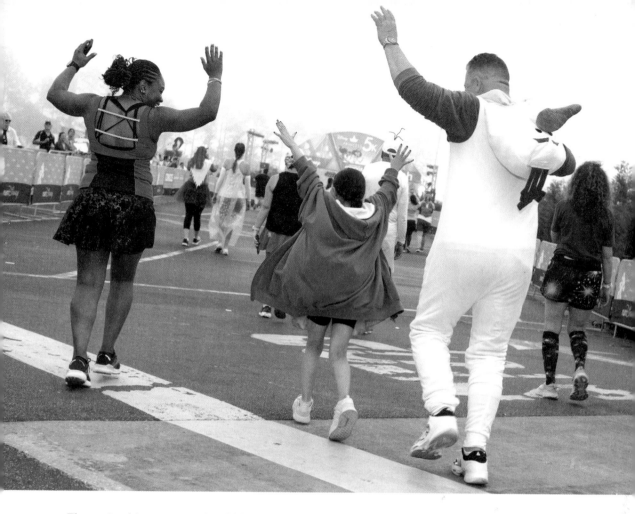

The main thing parents should keep in mind about running for anyone under eighteen is this: children should want to run, not be forced to run. If your child shows an interest in running, great. Help them nurture it. But if your child doesn't, accept it. Never pressure your child to run.

Even when your child shows an interest in running, it can be hard at first to determine whether it's genuine. They see how important running is to you, and they might want to please you by emulating what you do. On any given day, make sure your child is eager to run. Eventually, if it's not fun and they're primarily doing it because of you, they'll give it up. If that happens, don't tell them you're disappointed.

Fun should always be the guiding force in running—at any age. Most younger children don't yet grasp the concept of long-term goals. Their running should be about pleasure in the moment much more than results-driven motivations. (Come to think of it, that's not a bad outlook for adults!) Even teens shouldn't be encouraged to think about their running beyond the near future. And if your teen sets a running goal but then loses interest in it, that's fine. Kids these days already have too many have-tos in their lives.

Set up your child's runs so that it's easy for them to end at any time. Do loops around a field or the neighborhood, or go to a track. Don't fret about stopping at any point, either momentarily or for good. Monitor your child to make sure they're not breathing too hard. Stop the run immediately if they're limping or in obvious pain. At all times, run ever so slightly behind, even if you're running side by side. Don't get out front and create pressure for your child to keep up.

At some point your child might express interest in doing a race. That's good! There's no evidence that training for a race will stunt their growth or otherwise harm them long-term development. Running is a natural, healthful activity. (Spending all day slumped over a phone and not exercising . . . that's another matter.) There's also no evidence that doing races as a child will lead to burnout. All of the contributors to this book started running as teens, and are healthy and enthusiastic runners decades later.

Some runDisney events feature a slate of races for children nine or younger. See chapter 6 for details on those races. Kids and teens can also take part in the longer runDisney races, depending on their age. Here are the age requirements:

😈 5K: 5 and older.

😈 10K: 10 and older.

😈 10-Miler: 12 and older

😈 Half Marathon: 14 and older.

😈 Marathon: 18 and older.

The same principles apply to children who run races as it does to children who run in general: the child should be self-motivated. Your support should take the form of making sure they're enjoying it, and being okay with them not doing the race if their interest wanes.

While fun should always underlie your child's race training, you want to make sure they're ready to have a pleasurable experience on race day. Use the official runDisney training programs or other respected training programs. A young runner can usually gut their way through a distance they're unprepared for, but that's no way to

start what could be a lifetime sport and activity.

Training for a race shouldn't consume your child's life. They should stay on top of schoolwork, friendships, and other activities that they enjoy. They should keep growing while training, and should lose little to no weight. You can do your part by providing good nutrition and encouraging good sleep habits.

Come race day, let your child set the pace. Keep the emphasis on fun and participation. And don't forget your phone—you're going to want to document this moment.

A final point: Be a good ambassador for running! Model your love of running around your children. Through your words and actions, subtly show how much better your life is because of running. Give your children the gift of a good example.

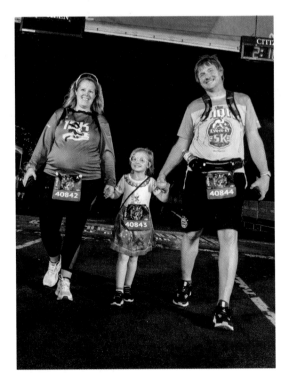

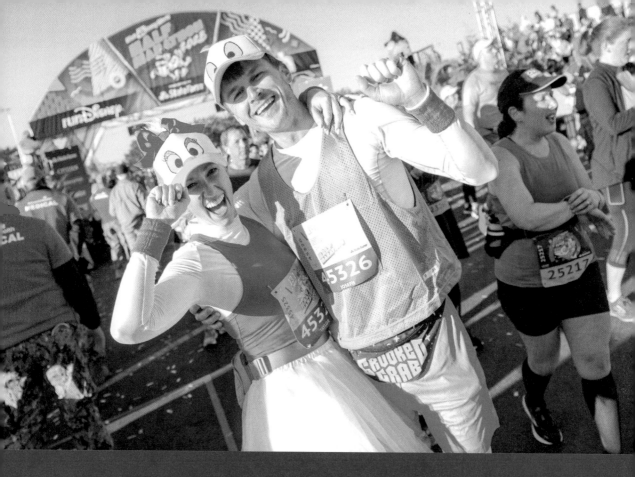

CHAPTER 8:
RUNNING WITH DISNEY STYLE

Do you want to stand out at a runDisney event? Then run in straightforward, everyday running apparel.

You'll be in the minority dressed like that. Running in some form of a Disney character costume is the norm, though, of course, not mandatory! It's been that way from the first runDisney race in 1994 . . . and gets more popular every year.

(Hello, social media!) You will never feel more at home as a Disney fan than when running amid thousands of others showcasing their Disney style.

In this chapter, we'll take a quick look at how to create your costume and what to expect when running in it.

GETTING IN CHARACTER

There are lots of places to find ideas for building your runDisney character costume. Generally, runners are inspired by the event's weekend themes, and the hero characters of the weekend. If you'll be running with friends and family, consider creating group costumes based on these themes.

Don't feel bound to be overly literal in dreaming up your costume. Feel free to use the themes and hero characters as starting points and see where your imagination takes you.

Disney's social channels are a great place to see runners dressed up before, during, and after runDisney events. (You do follow runDisney on Instagram and Facebook, right?) The runDisney blog has some step-by-step costume-building content. Fan-created posts on Pinterest and YouTube are also popular sources of costume inspiration.

Most runDisney costumes are created in the style of what's become known as DisneyBounding. It's a way of dressing to suggest a character without trying to precisely emulate it. Outside of running, people wear their regular clothes when DisneyBounding, and add a few elements or accessories to evoke the image of the character. It's a more flexible approach than creating an exact-to-the letter character impersonation, which is known as cosplay (a mash-up of "costume" and "play").

DisneyBounding makes good sense for runDisney events. For starters, cosplaying could conflict with one or more of the official runDisney guidelines for running in character. For example, donning a full Darth Vader costume would mean wearing a mask (not allowed) and a full-length cape (another no-no).

In addition, DisneyBounding gives you the freedom to make your character costume as extravagant or minimalist as you want. You'll want to strike a balance between full-character representation and representing your character while running several miles. As we'll cover, running in costume can present challenges—otherwise known as sweating and chafing—that don't really come up and distract when following DisneyBound pursuits in a more leisurely way.

DisneyBounding also means you don't have to be a wizard at the sewing machine to make a great costume. You might already own most of the clothing you'll need for a great running costume. After all, runners are no strangers to activewear skirts and leggings. Don't get too hung up on exactly matching the colors associated with a given character. If you have light green leggings instead of pea-green tights, nobody's going to dis your Peter Pan costume. And certainly don't set aside your tried-and-true running shoes just because another pair is a spot-on color match.

If your current running wardrobe won't quite satisfy the look you're going for, you don't have to spend a fortune to complete an outfit. Thrift shops are a great source for gently used athletic gear and costume accessories. Most running stores and online running merchants offer deep discounts on prior seasons' gear. You can get a swath or two of cloth at a fabric store to make accents for your costume. Craft stores are full of do-it-yourself goodies that can be helpful, such as color dyes that you can apply to clothes you already own.

Many DisneyBounders use accessories to take their costumes up a notch. Bracelets, necklaces, and earrings with the right design can stand in for larger items associated with a character. This approach is an especially good idea for running in costume, to lighten your mobile load.

RUNDISNEY COSTUME GUIDELINES

Fun and safety are the watchwords for all things runDisney—and that includes running in costume. So, while it's your adventure, and everyone at a runDisney event can dress as their favorite characters, there are some rules of the road.

- Costumes must be family-friendly, and can't be obstructive, offensive, objectionable, or evoke violence.

- Costumes can't contain sharp objects, pointed objects, or materials that might accidentally strike another runner.

- Costumes can't include toy weapons that resemble or could easily be mistaken for an actual weapon. For example, metal swords aren't permitted, but foam swords are.

- For runners fourteen and older, masks aren't allowed. That's the case even if the mask covers only part of your face, and regardless of whether your eyes are covered.

- For runners thirteen and younger, masks are allowed, if the mask doesn't cover the entire face (and if the eyes are visible).

- Hats and other headwear are allowed if they don't cover your face.

- Costumes can't reach or drag on the ground (like full-length Princess dresses do).

- Capes may be worn if they don't extend below your waist.

- Themed T-shirts, blouses, sweatshirts, and hats are acceptable.

- Acceptable accessories include transparent wings, plastic lightsabers, toy swords, and tutus.

- Layered costumes that could conceal prohibited items aren't allowed.

- Costume props, including those that surround your entire body, aren't permitted.

- If you're dressed as a Disney character, you can't pose for pictures or sign autographs for other guests.

- No costumed attire can be worn in Disney theme parks during operating hours. Bring a change of clothes to put on before visiting the parks once your race is over.

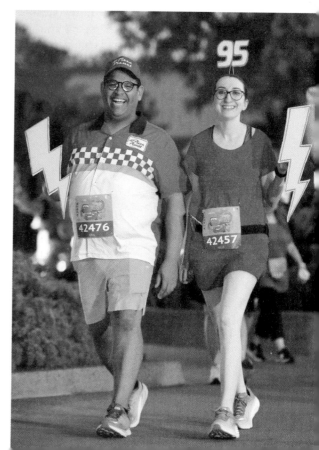

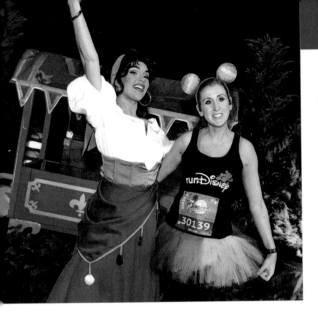

🐭 Guests who don't adhere to these guidelines may be refused entry into and/or removed from a race or any race-related event/activity unless their costume can be modified to meet the cited standards. It's better to plan ahead and make sure your costume meets the guidelines stipulated here than having to miss out on any of the fun.

🐭 Disney reserves the right to deny admission to or remove any person wearing attire that it considers inappropriate or attire that could detract from the experience of other guests.

HOW TO BE THE CONSUMMATE COSTUME RUNNER

Maximize your fun by following these tips before and during your runDisney costume adventure.

KEEP AN OPEN MIND: Treat costume running choice as one more way to make your running enjoyable. People run races for all sorts of reasons. Just as having variety in your training day to day, week to week, and month to month brings the best results, varying your mental approach to running throughout the year will keep you fresher. If for you that means running as your favorite Disney character, go for it. There are thousands of other races where donning a costume in a race isn't the norm; so why not save your standard running gear for those?

Don't worry about whether others might think you're not a "real runner" (whatever that means) because you're going to do a race in a costume. Women and men have run sub-3:00 marathons in costumes more often than many realize, so obviously there's no conflict between fun and fast. Who knows what future runners you'll inspire to take up the sport when they see a beloved character run past having the time of his or her life?

DO SOME PRACTICE RUNS: No matter how fast you plan to run in costume, you want it to be an enjoyable experience. The running wisdom of "Never try anything new on race day" certainly applies here. Halfway through a half marathon isn't the time to learn that your costume literally rubs you the wrong way.

Do one or two practice runs in costume to see what's likely to result in terms of chafing, pieces

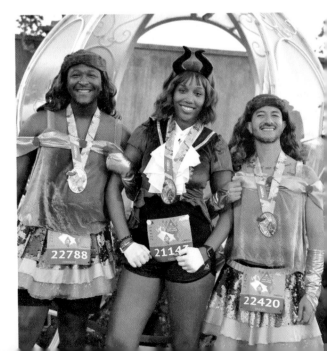

WHAT A CAST OF CHARACTERS!

Like we said, costumed runners are the norm, not the exception, at runDisney races. Who are you most likely to see striding alongside you? That varies by the weekend, but overall, here are the most popular costumes. Feel free to choose from this list, or run as a different character and start a new trend.

THE CLASSICS:
- Mickey Mouse
- Minnie Mouse

- Donald Duck
- Goofy
- Ariel
- Jasmine and Aladdin
- Tinker Bell
- Aurora/Sleeping Beauty
- Cinderella and Prince Charming
- Pluto
- Belle and the Beast
- Tweedledee and Tweedledum

FROM THE MOVIES:
- Buzz Lightyear
- Woody

- Stormtroopers
- Princess Leia
- Han Solo
- Rey
- Darth Vader
- Kylo Ren

FROM ELSEWHERE IN THE WIDE WORLD OF DISNEY:
- Theme park inspirations, such as popular attractions and icons.
- Cast members, such as ice cream scoopers and PhotoPass photographers.

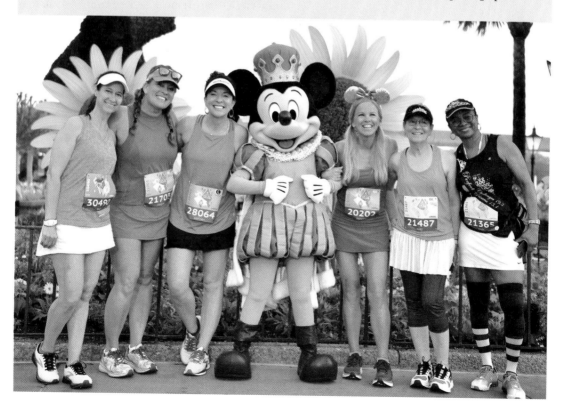

of costume staying in place, how much you sweat, and other costume-related matters. Keep these runs on the short side. Some of the materials in your costume probably weren't designed with distance running in mind. Going too far prerace might damage your costume. Just go far enough to make sure it fits, stays on, and doesn't have any obvious sources of irritation.

Bonus: your test runs might well become events in themselves. Certainly, the neighborhood children will appreciate seeing you in action this way. If you're getting ready for one or more races at the Walt Disney World Marathon Weekend in January, might we suggest doing a costume test run on Halloween?

EXPECT CHALLENGES: Practice runs will provide you an idea of what you're likely to encounter, but won't necessarily give you all the details.

Depending on what you wear, the biggest challenge could come from sweating more than usual. You'll want to be sure to pay extra attention to hydration before and during costume races, particularly those that are 10K and longer. Lots of sweating might also cause chafing when navigating the later miles. Apply a lubricant in potential problem areas prerace. Also consider cutting a few holes in your costume to allow more heat to escape. If chafing does occur, tell yourself you knew it was a possibility, and keep going.

Before your race, work through what extra logistics might be involved if you need to take a bathroom break en route.

Because masks aren't allowed at runDisney events, you'll be spared figuring out how to breathe through a small mouth hole.

EXPECT CHEERS: You're that rare costume runner if you're not at least a little interested in getting a reaction from others. And there's nothing wrong with that!

Costume running a runDisney event is a little different than doing so in other road races. At runDisney, you'll be surrounded by others in costume. In other races, you're more likely to be one of a handful of costumed runners. But that doesn't mean you won't get recognized at runDisney. Expect to hear from your fellow runners, spectators, maybe even official Disney characters as you speed past.

We all need a little outside support during races. You can count on getting it when you do a costume run—especially at a runDisney race. And don't forget to return the favor—cheer on your favorite characters when you spot them near you.

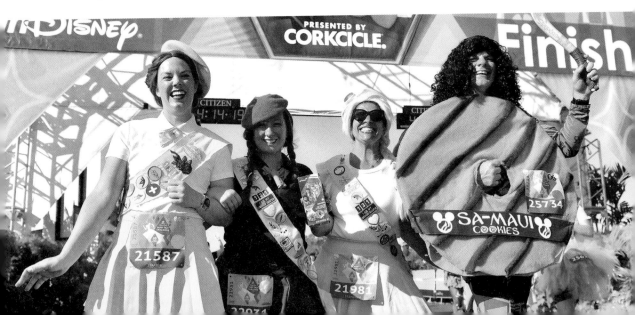

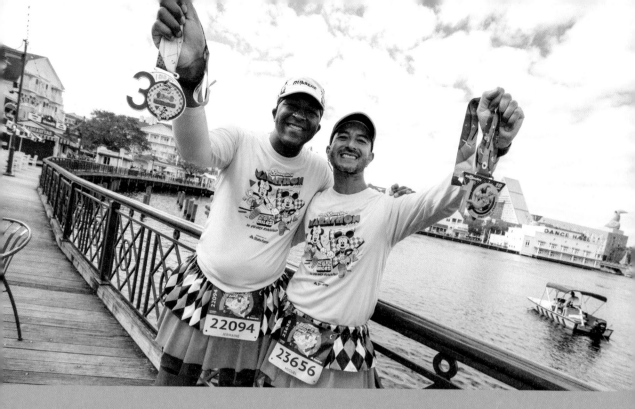

CHAPTER 9:
HOW TO CONQUER A RUNDISNEY CHALLENGE

We runners tend to have a more-is-better approach. That's especially true when fun, camaraderie, and celebration are on the menu. Every runDisney event includes at least one weekend challenge that involves running races on consecutive days. (See chapter 6 for a full description of the multiday challenges available throughout the runDisney season.)

Why do it? Why, for example, run the Disney Wine & Dine 10K on Saturday and the Disney Wine & Dine Half Marathon on Sunday to complete the Disney Two Course Challenge? Or why the Walt Disney World 5K on Thursday, Walt

Disney World 10K on Friday, Walt Disney World Half Marathon on Saturday, and the Walt Disney World Marathon on Sunday to complete the Dopey Challenge?

The best answer: Why not? Why not fully experience the runDisney magic?

Whatever your motivation, you can ensure you have a peak experience by putting a little extra thought into your training, how you run each race, and what you do between each challenge race you've committed yourself to. Let's look at how to master those aspects of a runDisney challenge.

TRAINING FOR YOUR CHALLENGE

It's easy to find guidance on training for stand-alone races. (Of course, we recommend the official runDisney programs available at rundisney.com.) How to train for running races taking place two or more days in a row is a different matter. Challenges such as those offered during runDisney weekends are rare in running circles. You've probably noticed that running, a weight-bearing sport, can produce more muscle soreness than other activities. That's probably why there's not a pro running equivalent of, say, cycling's Tour de France.

Don't panic—runDisney has you covered. The official runDisney training programs, created by

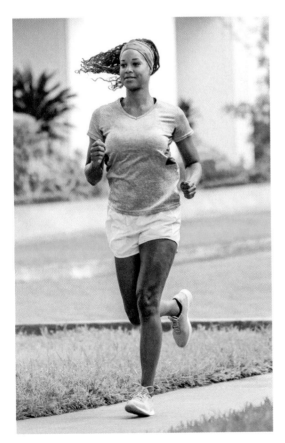

Olympian (and major contributor to this book) Jeff Galloway, include schedules for all of the runDisney challenges. For the challenges that combine a 10K on Saturday and a half marathon on Sunday, you'll find a nineteen-week program. There are twenty-nine-week training programs for the Goofy's Race and a Half Challenge (half marathon on Saturday, marathon on Sunday) and the Dopey Challenge.

All of the programs use the run-walk-run method to safely and gradually build your ability to cover a good distance on two or more consecutive days. We highly recommend that you consult the schedules even if you decide not to follow them exactly.

If you do devise your own training for your challenge, keep in mind the principle that underlies all good training programs: prepare your body and mind for the specific demands of your event.

You'll need to get used to running or run-walking on consecutive days. As your challenge approaches, you'll want to be getting near its longest distance on at least one of your consecutive-days training blocks.

Ideally, you'll do as is recommended in the runDisney challenge programs, and have that longest run be on the last day of your training blocks period. That simulates what you'll do during the challenge, with the race distance increasing throughout a runDisney race weekend. You'll also want to be able to do these training blocks relatively comfortably—dragging your way through each day won't set you up for a fun experience on race weekend.

If your schedule allows, do some of your training early in the morning. All the races start at 5:00 a.m. You'll enjoy your weekend a lot more if the race-day rise-and-run call isn't too big of a shock.

A FEW MORE TRAINING CONSIDERATIONS

Remember that all runDisney races require maintaining a pace of 16 minutes per mile or faster. You'll need to stay under that pace to earn your challenge medal. Check your pace occasionally on your longer runs. Be honest with yourself about whether you're ready to maintain a sub-16:00 mile pace as challenge weekend progresses and race distances increase.

Practice drinking and fueling on your longer training runs. Taking in liquids and, if you prefer, foods such as energy gels should be second nature by time you're doing a challenge weekend event. Experiment with the right amounts that keep you hydrated and fueled without upsetting your stomach or causing frequent pit stops. As we'll

see, it's more important to drink and eat during a challenge race event than it is during a stand-alone race.

The first four challenges in the runDisney season occur in January (Goofy's Race and a Half Challenge, Dumbo Double Dare Challenge, and the Dopey Challenge) and February (Disney Fairytale Challenge). If you're doing one of those and live where winters are cold, consider adding a little heat training to your preparation. Once or twice a week, run in extra clothes to simulate running in warmer conditions. Or do a couple of your long runs on a treadmill. You can also become more efficient at sweating by taking regular saunas.

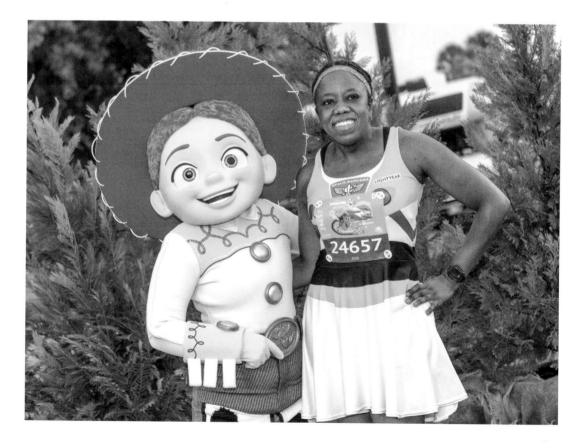

SLOW AND STEADY WINS THE MULTIDAY RACE EVENT

So, now it's challenge weekend. Disney will take care of the fun; you take care of yourself so that your weekend is a lifetime experience.

In terms of finishing your challenge relatively unscathed, there are two main things you can do: minimize damage to your body during each race, and accelerate the recovery process between races. Let's look first at what to do during each race, no matter the distance.

Proper pacing is always crucial to running your best races. It takes on a whole new level of importance when you're running two or more races on consecutive days. In a stand-alone race, if you start too fast, you'll suffer unnecessarily the second half of the run. But then it doesn't really matter how exhausted you are the following day. That doesn't apply, however, when you're doing a Disney challenge event. Pacing yourself poorly on that first day will mean you'll start the next day's race as slightly more damaged. And remember this: in all of the challenges, the race distance increases each day.

You'll also want to pace yourself in an overall sense. Say you're doing the Wine & Dine Challenge, with a 10K on Saturday and half marathon on Sunday. You could run the 10K at a perfectly even pace, but still not have paced yourself well. How so? If that perfectly even pace was fast enough to leave you as drained as a stand-alone 10K has. In other words, don't go as fast as you possibly can in any of the races before the last day of the challenge. It's okay to run strong, but that's different from making an all-out effort that leaves you spent.

If you want to try to complete your challenge at a pace that's faster than your normal training pace, there are a couple of smart ways to attempt this. You could start each race at an easy pace, and gradually speed up to your race pace for that distance by the second half of the race. So, if you're doing the Wine & Dine 10K on Saturday, you would start slow and build over the first 5K to your normal 10K race pace, and then hold that pace all the way to the finish. Alternatively, if you prefer to run the course at a more even pace, you could aim to run your 10-mile or half marathon pace for the 10K distance. That's a good solid pace that should still leave you ready to tackle the following day's half marathon.

Before deciding on your pacing strategy, check the dew point, which accounts for the combined effects of temperature and humidity. You can easily find local dew point readings on weather apps. If the dew point is 65 or higher, plan a more conservative pace from the start. You don't want to realize in the second half of any of the races that make up a runDisney happening that you've underestimated how draining the day's weather conditions are. The rest of your challenge will be less enjoyable if you have to push through dehydration one or more days.

With races at Walt Disney World Resort starting at 5:00 a.m., bright sun shouldn't be a concern except on half marathon and marathon days. Radiant heat from the sun will make you sweat more than the same temperature on an overcast day. You'll also want to apply sunscreen before any of the races you'll be running the bulk in after sunrise. You don't need to deal with a sunburn along with all of the miles on your plate.

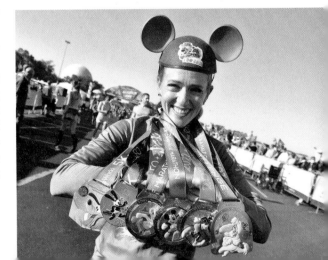

OTHER RACING CONSIDERATIONS

If you have more than one pair of running shoes, bring your two most comfortable, cushioned pairs. The second pair can be a backup in case something goes wrong with your usual go-to shoes, such as upper tearing in a shoe or the heel counter suddenly starting to cause friction. Your challenge shoes should be broken in some, ideally on at least a couple of long runs to confirm they'll work for you. But they shouldn't be nearing their end. You don't want to get halfway through your first race of the weekend and get that dead shoes/dead legs feeling.

Bring a couple of outfits that you've tested on long runs. (You might be fine with wearing the same running clothes a few sweaty days in a row, but your fellow racers will likely have other thoughts!) Minimize all potential sources of chafing and hot spots. Apply a lubricant to any body part where you've had chafing or irritation. Trim those gnarly runner toenails. It's one thing to have a little flesh wound when you don't plan to run the next day, but quite another when you have one or more races—and each one longer than the next—on ensuing days.

Stay adequately hydrated during each race. Your performance in an individual race can start to suffer once you become dehydrated by more than 2 percent of your body weight. If you weigh 160 pounds, that's 3.2 pounds, or roughly 1.5 liters of sweat. Getting too far past that level of dehydration will also significantly impede your recovery for your remaining races.

Remember from chapter 4 that "adequately hydrated" doesn't equal "as hydrated as possible." Only the most prolific sweaters will sweat out 2 percent of their weight during a 5K. A half marathon or marathon is a different matter. Drink enough to avoid feeling thirsty, but not so much that your stomach feels full and starts sloshing. You're better off drinking a small amount more frequently than stopping at two aid stations and chugging.

Fueling isn't really an issue in a 5K or 10K. In a half marathon or marathon, you'll want to take in some calories, in the form of liquid, energy gel, or other portable sport-nutrition offering. Doing so will help to preserve the energy stores of your muscles. And at least as important—the calories will keep your brain fed; you'll be more upbeat and alert, and a given pace will feel easier. Aim for 100 to 200 calories per 30 to 60 minutes, depending on how experienced you are with on-the-run fueling and how sensitive your stomach is. A typical energy gel contains about 100 calories.

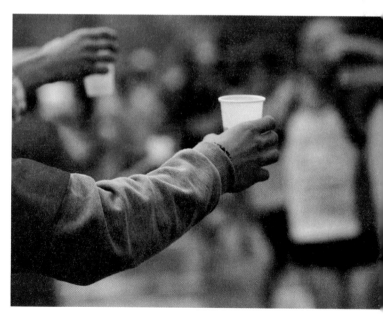

HOW TO MAXIMIZE RECOVERY BETWEEN RACES

Part of how you feel on day 2 (or 3, or 4) of your challenge depends on how you ran the day before. What you do after each day's race also plays a huge role in how rarin' to go you'll be the following morning. Here's how to get your body back to normal (or a reasonable semblance of normal) as quickly as possible.

IN THE FIRST HOUR AFTER FINISHING:

CHANGE CLOTHES. Your immune system is temporarily compromised after exercise. You'll be less likely to pick up a virus if you change into dry clothes. Plus, you'll feel and smell better!

KEEP MOVING. A gentle walk will maintain increased blood flow, which will help to remove waste products from your muscles and help your hormone levels return to resting levels sooner. As a result, by the afternoon you'll feel more like your prerace self than if you finish a race and sit down for fifteen minutes. You also won't be as sore for the next day's run.

After walking for ten to twenty minutes, do some gentle stretching while your muscles are still warm. You'll feel less creaky when you get up the next morning—and head out on the next challenge.

EAT AND DRINK. Continue to drink enough so that you're not thirsty. After a 10K or longer race, take in a few hundred calories as soon as it's feasible. Your body will restock its carbohydrate stores at a much higher rate the first thirty minutes after running, and the rate of storage remains elevated the first two hours after you've finished. A little protein within a carbohydrate-rich food or drink will speed along the restoring even more.

Plan for this postrace snack by having an energy bar or other easily portable item in your race-day bag. If your stomach is bothering you too much to eat, consume the calories in liquid form. Chocolate milk is a good simultaneous source of carbs and protein.

IN THE AFTERNOON:

EAT FOOD THAT WILL KEEP RESTOCKING YOUR MUSCLES. Foods with a higher glycemic index lead to larger increases in your blood glucose levels. That's a good thing in the few hours after finishing a race, because it will lead to more carbs being stored in your muscles for the following day's race. Some foods to emphasize at breakfast or lunch are rice, potatoes, bread products, fruit bars, crackers, and rice cakes. As with the immediate aftermath of your race, including a little protein will accelerate the process.

KEEP HYDRATING. Make sure you always have access to fluids. You don't want to find yourself suddenly thirsty and be without a chance to quench that thirst. As always, smaller, more frequent drinks will help you stay on top of hydration better than waiting until you're thirsty and drinking a lot at once.

KEEP YOUR MUSCLES LOOSE. Take a hot shower or bath when you get back to your room. Then, while your muscles are a little warmer, do some more gentle stretching or yoga. Pay special attention to any particularly tight spots. This is also a good time for gentle foam rolling or other forms of self-massage. The key word here is "gentle." You want to help any sore or tight spots loosen, not further aggravate them. Find that hurts-so-good/that's-the-spot amount of pressure, and then back off a little.

TEND TO ANY WAR WOUNDS. If you had chafing, a blister, a hot spot, or some other skin irritation during your race, treat the area so that it bothers you as little as possible the following morning.

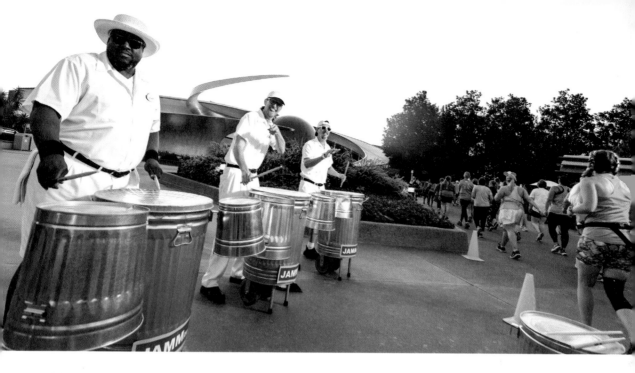

RELAX IN COMPRESSION GEAR. We saw in chapter 3 that compression gear is probably most effective when worn for recovery. Compression tights and knee-high socks should reduce feelings of muscle soreness and fatigue.

BEFORE GOING TO BED:

EAT A CARBOHYDRATE-RICH DINNER. Continuing to emphasize carbohydrates will ensure you start the following day's race fully fueled. Keep in mind that a carbohydrate-rich dinner doesn't mean to chow down on as much pasta as you can stomach. Too large of a dinner could interfere with your sleep and increase your chances of a mid-race pit stop the following morning. If you did a good job of refueling throughout the day after your race, there's no reason to eat more than your normal portion sizes for dinner. Just make sure those portions contain a lot of carbs.

EAT DINNER ON THE EARLY SIDE. You'll be getting up early the next morning. Digestion and feeling full can get in the way of falling asleep.

KEEP HYDRATING. Ideally, you'll have done a stellar job during the day and through dinner at avoiding thirst. If by dinnertime your urine is about the color of straw, you should be set. Downing large amounts of liquid after dinner will probably interrupt your sleep, since you'll have to make frequent trips to the bathroom.

BE CAREFUL WITH CAFFEINE AND ALCOHOL. Forgo coffee and caffeinated tea by late afternoon. Yes, you might be dragging a little before dinner because of getting up early and racing. But the price to pay for any temporary pickup will likely be compromised sleep. One or two drinks (say a twelve-ounce beer or glass of wine) shouldn't interfere too much with your sleep if that's something you're used to.

SET YOURSELF UP FOR GOOD SLEEP. Try not to use your phone or view other kinds of screens within the hour before you want to go to sleep. The blue light from these devices stalls the release of melatonin, a hormone that signals to your body to start falling asleep.

Don't force yourself to go to bed if you're not feeling sleepy. Lying down should signal to your body that it's time to sleep. Lying in bed worrying that you're not falling asleep does more harm than good.

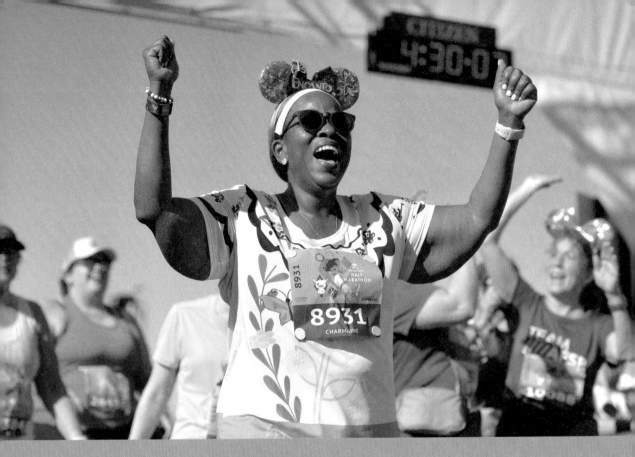

CHAPTER 10:
MAINTAINING THE MAGIC

You did it! You ran a runDisney race (or two or three) and had a magical weekend. Now's it time to. . . . what?

Well, that's a good question. What happens now that your runDisney weekend is behind you?

It's natural after a big event or achieving a momentous goal to feel a little adrift. This thing in the future you've been building up to for so long is now in the past. Fortunately, because of your runDisney experience, you have the perfect tool for figuring out what's next: go for a run and think things through.

In this final chapter, we'll look at ways to keep running fun for a long, long time. You'll want to read it whether you've done one runDisney event, a dozen, or none. Because who doesn't want to keep having fun?

RIGHT AFTER YOUR RACE

First things first: It's celebration time. And what better place to celebrate at than a Disney Park? Go crazy with the rides and entertainment now that you're not worried about getting tired before your next race. If you were being super careful about what you were eating in the days before your race, now's the time to let your cravings dictate the menu.

Don't feel bad about sharing your accomplishment with others. Friends and family back home and on your social media feeds will want to know how it went, and what it looked like. Wear your race shirt and medal around the resort. Tell people what a great time you had. Maybe you'll inspire them to start running so that they can get in on the runDisney magic.

Use the immediate aftermath of your race as a time to savor your experience. A couple of days later, when the emotions and excitement of the moment have passed, do a debriefing with yourself. Review your training for the race. What worked well? What didn't pan out? What did you learn that you can incorporate into your future running?

Then do the same sort of analysis for your race. What did you do well? What were the highlights? What are the areas where you could have been better? Did those things happen because of something you did in your preparation for the race, or because of something that happened during the race?

You'll have time to ponder and reflect on things soon after your race, because if you're smart, you'll take a few days off from running. Even the best runners in the world often take a short break from running right after a big race. (Or not so short, if they've run a marathon.) A few days off from running won't mean that you'll suddenly get out of shape. They'll help your body recover from your race and the training you did leading up to it.

It's not a sign of weakness—or evidence that you're not really a runner—if you enjoy these days off. Do things around the house, stay up late, sleep in, catch up with friends, do whatever you want that you may have had to set aside a bit while training for your race. Don't worry about running again until you start to feel antsy. That's a sign that your body and mind are eager to get going again. If you have that feeling but your body is still sore or tight enough that you can't run with your normal form, go for a walk, ride a bike, or find some other form of exercise that won't leave you in more pain.

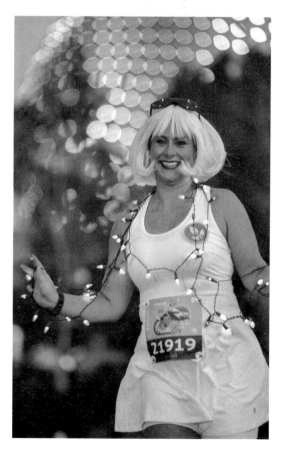

FIGURING OUT THE FUTURE

Way back in chapter 1, we saw how having good goals makes your running easier and more enjoyable. You know what you want to do and what you need to do to get there. Now that you've met one runDisney goal, it's time to figure out what's next.

Your new goal doesn't have to be something you must get to work on right away. Immediately after your race, you're in recovery mode. But take this time to do some thinking. What will motivate you going forward? What's something else that you get fired up about when you think about it? What brings out a smile when you imagine yourself accomplishing it?

Remember, too, that good goals have a time element. You think not only *I want to do X*, but also tell yourself when you'll do it. In the case of a race, especially a runDisney event, that time element is more or less picked for you. That set-in-stone date—sorry, they're running the race even if you're not there—can make things easier. You know when you need to be ready; now you just need to plan how to get ready.

It's completely fine to set a goal that's quite far in the future. Maybe you just got back from doing the half marathon at the Walt Disney World Marathon Weekend gathering. The day after the half marathon, you watched the marathon and told yourself you want to join in and extend the fun. That means your goal is a year away. There's nothing wrong with that. Under this scenario, you could block out the several months before the marathon as your key training time, and in the interim have as your goal something like this: *Until marathon training starts, maintain the fitness I built training for the half marathon.*

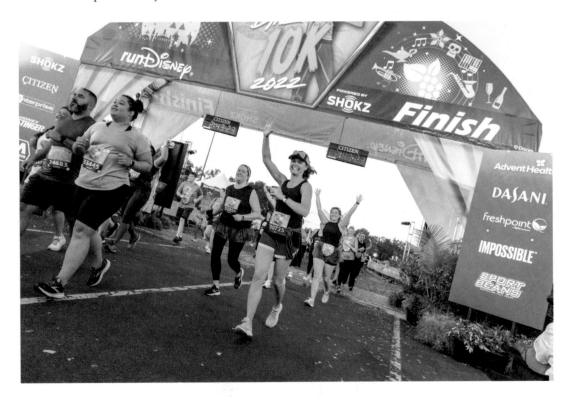

WHERE SHOULD THE MAGIC STRIKE NEXT?

Let's say you just finished a runDisney race. One approach when looking toward the future is to go back and see what you can do there again. Many people cherish the objectivity of running. It's satisfying to see that you ran a certain time at, say, the Disney Wine & Dine 10K one year, and then a year later returned to finish the same course faster. Running can provide black-and-white feedback that can be difficult to match in other parts of your life.

Another approach is to, well . . . take a different approach. Consider these other ways to experience the runDisney magic:

TRY A DIFFERENT DISTANCE: Once you've conquered one distance, it's natural to think about going farther. Can you follow up that 5K finisher medal with one for a 10K? Can you go more than twice as far as you did in the 10K and finish a half marathon? And once you've nailed a half marathon, are you ready to take on the fabled marathon?

TRY A DIFFERENT PACE: Instead of moving up in race distance, how about moving down? Now that you know you can run a half marathon, why not see just how fast you can run a 5K or 10K? Focusing on a shorter distance doesn't make you less of a runner. Doing so will make you a more well-rounded runner, and if you eventually return to longer races, you'll have a new degree of speed that will help you at any distance.

TRY A DIFFERENT EMPHASIS: All races are fun, no matter how you run them. But it's easy to get in a routine where you have the same general approach for each one. Consider mixing things up! Run your next runDisney race as a group with family and friends. Run for charity. See how many high fives you can get per mile. Run in a costume. Pace a friend to her first 5K finish. There are infinite ways to experience a race. Be creative about how you do so the next time.

TRY A VIRTUAL RACE: You might not be able to get to a Disney resort for your next race, but you can still race the runDisney way. Do one or more of the virtual races described in chapter 6. You set the date, time, and course, so you can race when and where you'll most be ready to shine. And you'll still get a themed finisher's medal.

TRY A DIFFERENT THEME: If you had a great time at one runDisney event, you're certainly welcome to come back the following year. But how about choosing a different weekend? New themes, new costumes, new heroes, new time of year? Not only will the weekend itself be different, but so will your buildup, because you'll be training in a different season than last time.

TRY A CHALLENGE: Surely your interest in trying a runDisney challenge has been piqued. What better way is there than to celebrate your love of running and Disney? Enough said!

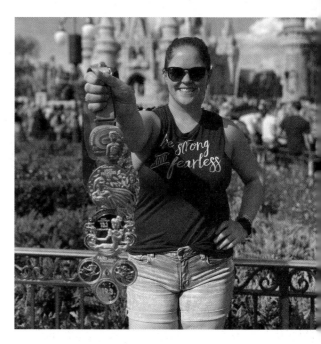

IN THE LONG RUN

The best running goal of all? To always be a runner. Here are some parting thoughts on how to make that happen.

STAY HEALTHY: Keeping your body able to do what you want it to do really is the key to fulfilling long-term joy in running. To reiterate a crucial point from chapter 5, consider regular strengthening and stretching exercises as being as much a part of being a runner as running itself.

A good way to make doing a few minutes of these exercises an integral part of your life most days is to set a goal such as "miss no days of running due to injury in the next six months." That goal doesn't mean that you run regardless of whether you're hurt. It's a way to provide daily

motivation for doing your supplementary exercises; you can tell yourself you're doing them to help you meet your goal. Eventually, doing the exercises won't seem like a chore, because you'll feel worse running when you don't do them regularly.

STAY OPEN-MINDED: Always be open to new aspects of running. There are innumerable ways to be a runner. You don't have to actively explore them all, but why automatically shut yourself off from them? If some aspect of running speaks to you, pursue it.

Don't worry about what others think of your various versions of being a runner. Your running is for you, not them. Maybe the harshest critic

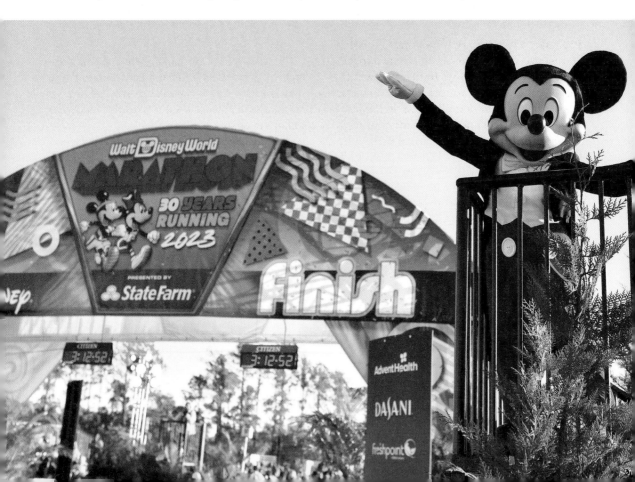

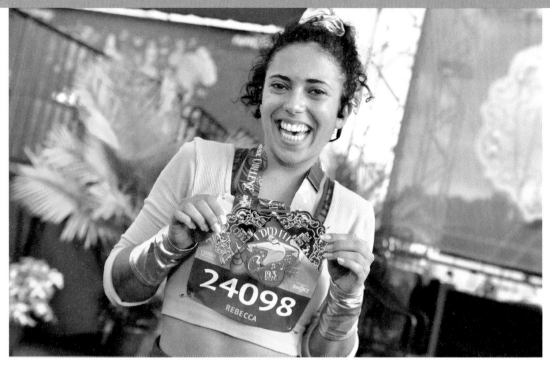

you'll face when you try something new will be a younger version of yourself. Tell that younger self that, as in so many things in life, that was then, this is now. Just because road half marathons once called to you doesn't mean you're a lesser runner if they don't now. The important thing is to keep running.

STAY SOCIAL: One of the great pleasures of running is how it paves the way to socializing with others; it's built into its fabric. At races and on training runs, you can nurture existing friendships and form new ones. You'll want to keep running just so you can keep up—literally and figuratively—with your friends.

Running will introduce you to people of all ages and backgrounds. You would never get to know most of these people otherwise. Sharing some miles with them will build bonds that will be deeper and more intimate than the ways most other activities offer. While many of your contemporaries see their social circles shrink with age, yours can become larger and more diverse every year that you keep running.

STAY SANE: We saw in chapter 2 the training principle of "hurry slowly." That mix of ambition and patience is crucial to making progress as a runner. Writ large, it's also a good way to go about your long-term approach to running.

Always strive to keep your running in perspective. That's another way of saying to make your approach to running sustainable over the long haul. Find ways to weave running into the fabric of your life so that it's a normal part of your schedule. At the same time, avoid making running so dominant that it gets in the way of the other important parts of your life. That's not going to work out well for anyone over the years and, hopefully, the decades of running ahead of you.

STAY FUN: Finding pleasure and meaning in your running underlies all the points and issues covered. Running will vastly improve your quality of life if you don't turn it into just another obligation. You already have enough of those.

Whether you're at a runDisney event or elsewhere, keep your running magical!

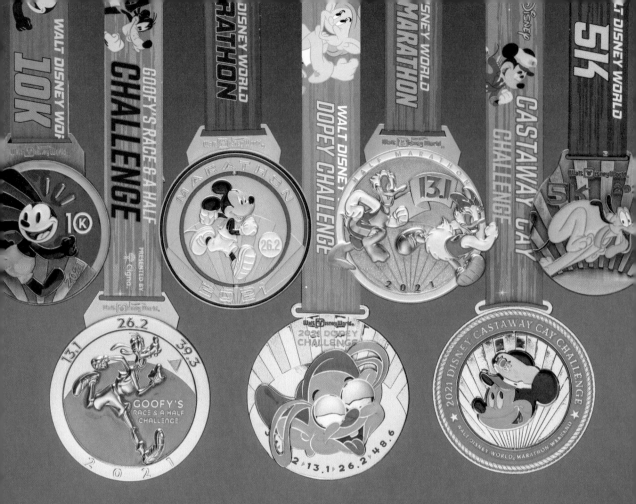

CHAPTER 11
A GALLERY
OF MEDALS

Enthusiastic collectors find the search just as rewarding as the discovery. And never more so than with runDisney fans. The race medals, featured here in detail, are the holy grail for collectors. The journey to acquiring them is the most fun of all. Spending time training and getting ready for races and then spending weekends enjoying the fitness benefits of running are the perfect combination to continue to add to your collection.

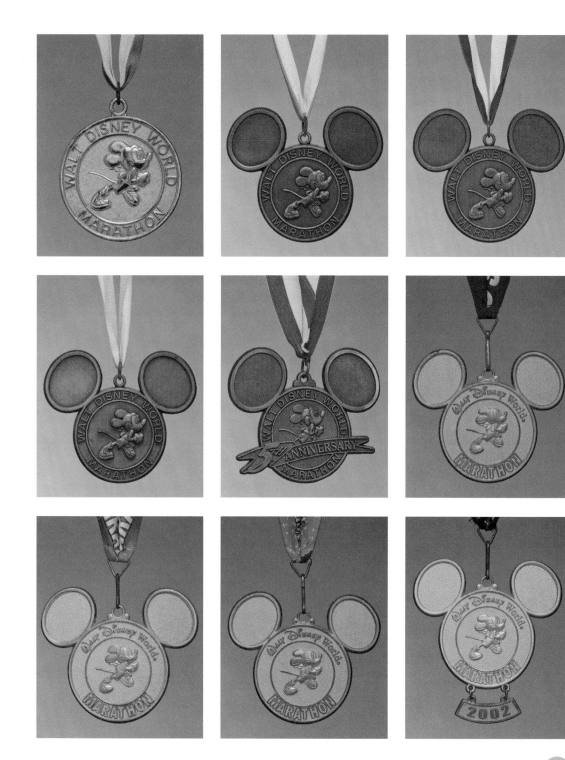

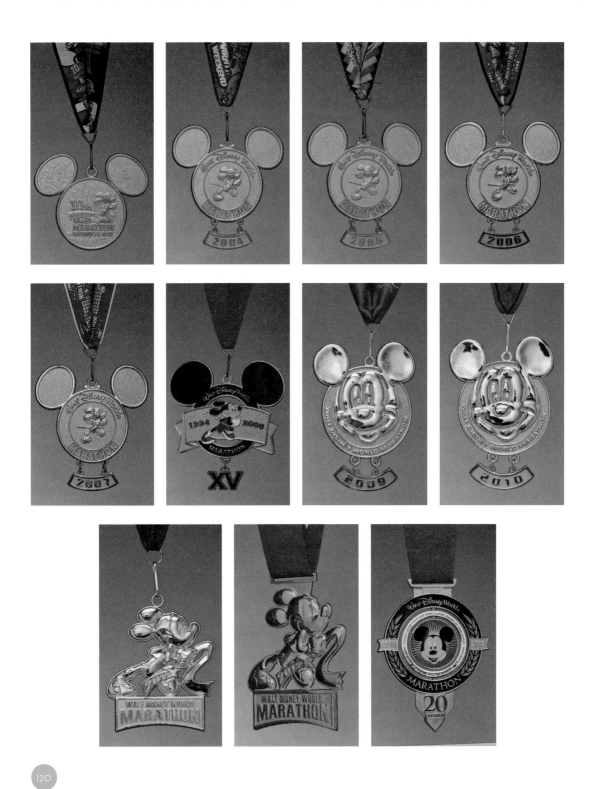

2014

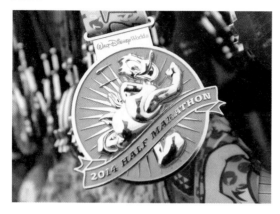
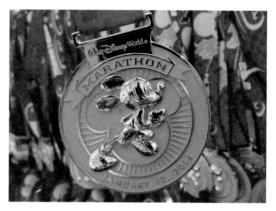

2015

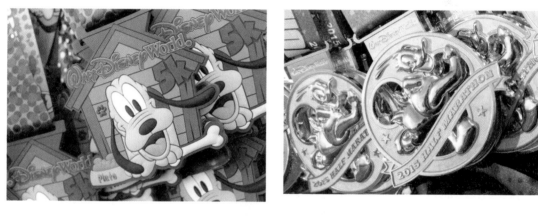

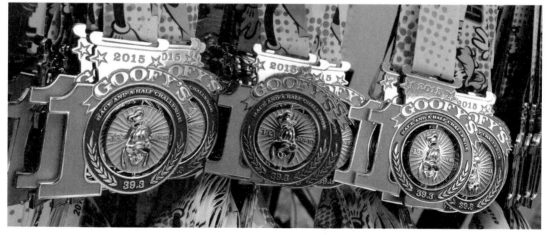

2016

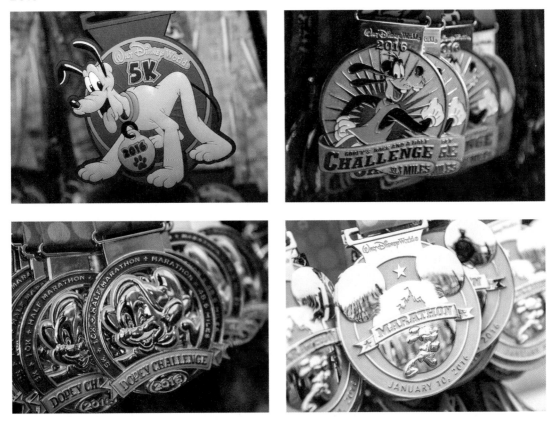

2017

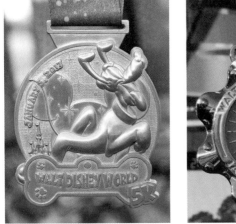

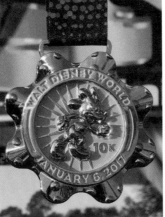

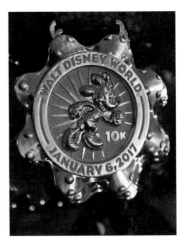

2018

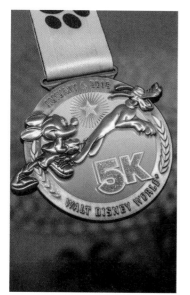

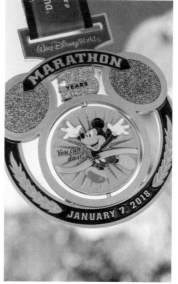

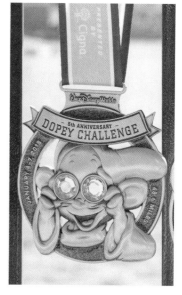

2019

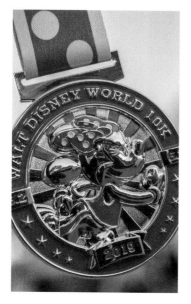

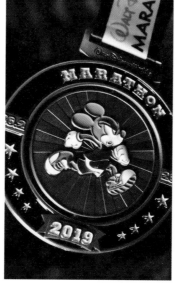

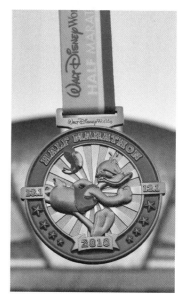

2020

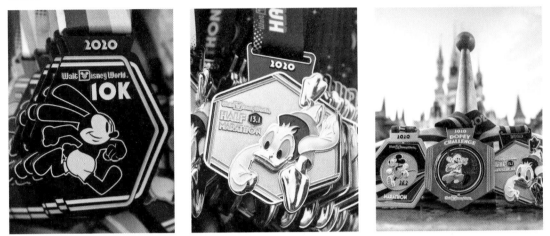

2021

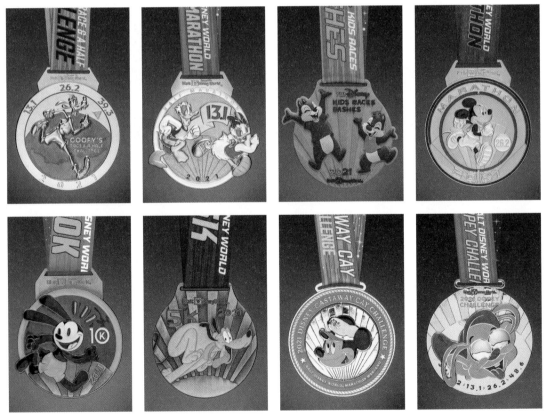

2022

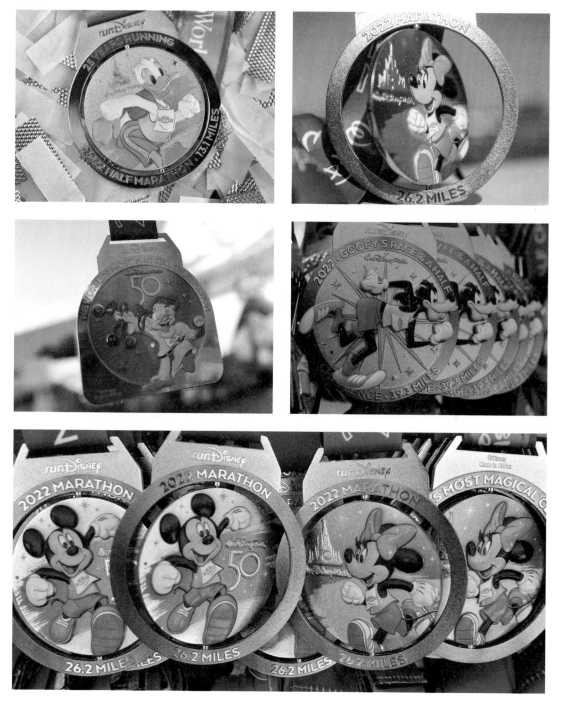

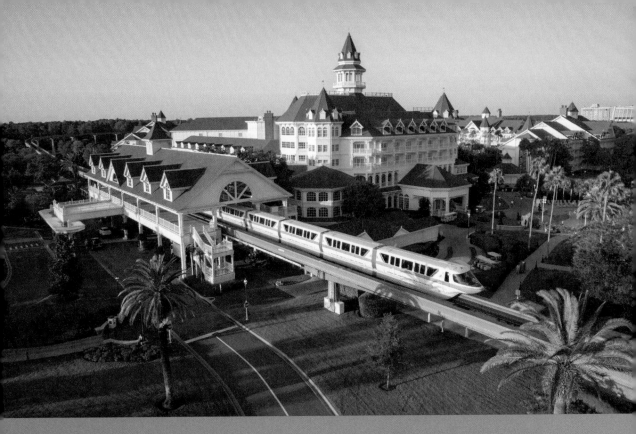

APPENDIX:
WALT DISNEY WORLD AND DISNEYLAND RESORTS

MAGIC KINGDOM AREA RESORTS

DISNEY'S CONTEMPORARY RESORT

This resort is perfect for both families and professionals. The monorail goes right through the resort, and the Magic Kingdom is only steps away. There are also fun character meals at Chef Mickey's.

DISNEY'S FORT WILDERNESS CABINS AND CAMPGROUND RESORT

Perfect for seasoned RV enthusiasts and guests who appreciate the modern amenities of the cabins, this resort also features pony and wagon rides, plus a nightly campfire circle with Chip and Dale.

DISNEY'S GRAND FLORIDIAN RESORT & SPA

Manicured rose gardens and a beautiful, romantic atmosphere are the hallmarks of this resort. There's also a Mad Hatter–themed splash zone for the kids.

DISNEY'S POLYNESIAN VILLAGE RESORT

This property has a real resort feel, with lush tropical settings and beach swings for two. The lava pool (with its decorative volcano motif) has a slide and waterfall. And you can get a Dole Whip at Pineapple Lanai, or dine with Lilo and Stitch at 'Ohana.

DISNEY'S WILDERNESS LODGE

Here's a great option for summer, as well as winter (when the warm and cozy atmosphere is made even more inviting since the fireplace in the lobby is roaring). Plus, its Story Book Dining at Artist Point offers guests an exclusive chance to meet the Queen from *Snow White*.

EPCOT AREA RESORTS

DISNEY'S BOARDWALK INN

Guests who love EPCOT and want more entertainment options at night will love the BoardWalk Inn. And kids will love the Keister Coaster, a two-hundred-foot-long waterslide at the main pool.

DISNEY'S CARIBBEAN BEACH RESORT

Families love the colorful rooms, pirate-themed pool, and secluded beach setting. There's access to the Disney Skyliner.

DISNEY'S RIVIERA RESORT

A rooftop restaurant at this resort offers prime views of theme park fireworks shows, plus there are peaceful strolls to be had around the nearby Barefoot Bay.

DISNEY'S YACHT & BEACH CLUB RESORTS

The central location of these two resorts offers easy access for those who want to try everything at WDW, plus a great pool, Stormalong Bay. EPCOT fans also enjoy the proximity to that park.

DISNEY SPRINGS AREA RESORTS

DISNEY'S OLD KEY WEST RESORT

Guests looking for a homey, village atmosphere will love this resort. Private whirlpool tubs come with all accommodations, except at the studios.

DISNEY'S PORT ORLEANS RESORT

With peaceful gardens scattered about the Riverside quarters, this resort also delivers gorgeous interior décor, and easy boat access to Disney Springs. The French Quarter, meanwhile, provides a peaceful, urban environment with a sea serpent-themed family pool.

DISNEY'S SARATOGA SPRINGS RESORT & SPA

Pretty gardens and meandering pathways are the hallmarks of this resort. Private whirlpool tubs are in all the property's accommodations—except the studios.

ANIMAL KINGDOM AREA RESORTS

DISNEY'S ALL-STAR MOVIES, MUSIC, AND SPORTS RESORT

Great for anyone who may be watching their budget, these resorts offer fun, colorful theming, and all of the Walt Disney World perks, but at a lower price than many other Disney resorts.

DISNEY'S ANIMAL KINGDOM LODGE

Here's a practically perfect resort for animal lovers. Guests can book Savanna View rooms, which afford amazing views of wandering wildlife. There are also delicious and unique dining options.

DISNEY'S CORONADO SPRINGS RESORT

Guests can enjoy the unique blend of Spanish, Mexican, and Southwest American cultures celebrated at Coronado Springs.

ESPN WIDE WORLD OF SPORTS AREA RESORTS

DISNEY'S ART OF ANIMATION RESORT

This popular resort has one of the nicest food courts in all of Walt Disney World. The family suites can accommodate up to six people, so they are perfect for extended families (or families with babies). There's also easy access to the Skyliner.

DISNEY'S POP CENTURY RESORT

With a state-of-the-art arcade and daily dance parties at the food court, this resort is perfect for nostalgia buffs who are watching their budget. Pop Century also features access to the Disney Skyliner.

NON-DISNEY-OWNED DISNEY SPRINGS RESORT AREA HOTELS

B RESORT & SPA

This resort has all of the modern amenities, including 47-inch HD flat-screen TVs, bunk beds (in select rooms), iPad docking stations, and kitchenettes in the suites. There is also a heated outdoor infinity-edge saltwater pool and a full-service spa and wellness center.

DOUBLETREE SUITES BY HILTON

The only all-suite hotel in the Disney Springs area, the property includes a heated pool and whirlpool, as well as a splash pad and a playground for kids. There's also a newly updated fitness center and a Disney shop.

FOUR SEASONS ORLANDO

This 443-room luxury property boasts more than twenty-six lakeside acres of elegant design. The resort features complimentary transportation to the theme parks and Disney character breakfasts on Thursdays and Saturdays. Guest rooms come with furnished balconies, DVD players, terrycloth robes, and minibars.

HILTON BUENA VISTA PALACE

The tallest hotel in the Disney Springs area, this resort has numerous modern amenities, including Wi-Fi, flat-screen TVs, and a pool bar and restaurant. Most rooms also have either a balcony or patio.

HILTON ORLANDO LAKE BUENA VISTA

The resort offers two heated outdoor pools, a splash pad for kids, and a steak house that serves sushi. Guests also have access to the Skybridge, a raised walkway that connects to Disney Springs across the street.

HOLIDAY INN

This family-friendly hotel features a restaurant, a heated pool, a whirlpool, and a Disney Store. There is also a twenty-four-hour fitness center and a twenty-four-hour game room.

WYNDHAM

This resort offers two distinct lodging options: one's a nineteen-story tower with 232 rooms known as the Wyndham Lake Buena Vista; the other one is in the Wyndham Garden section, which holds 394 rooms. They are spread over two five-story buildings.

PROPERTIES IN THE DISNEYLAND RESORT

DISNEYLAND HOTEL

With its monorail-themed pool—complete with waterslides—and light-up Sleeping Beauty Castle headboards, this resort has a nostalgic yet modern appeal. It is within walking distance to Downtown Disney and both theme parks, and features a wide array of dining options, including Goofy's Kitchen.

DISNEY'S GRAND CALIFORNIAN HOTEL & SPA

Recently refurbished, this four-star hotel takes the form of a modern art gallery that has assembled the Earth's mightiest Marvel artwork. Amenities include extra magic time at the parks, free shuttle to the parks, a generous breakfast buffet, and more.

PIXAR PLACE HOTEL

Formerly known as the Paradise Pier Hotel, this resort has recently undergone a massive transformation. Familiar friends from *Toy Story*; *Monsters, Inc.*; and other Pixar films make families feel at home here—as does the *Finding Dory* splash pad.

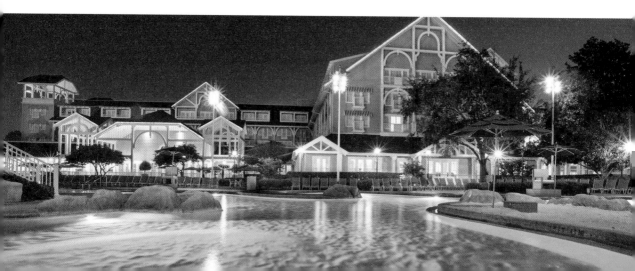

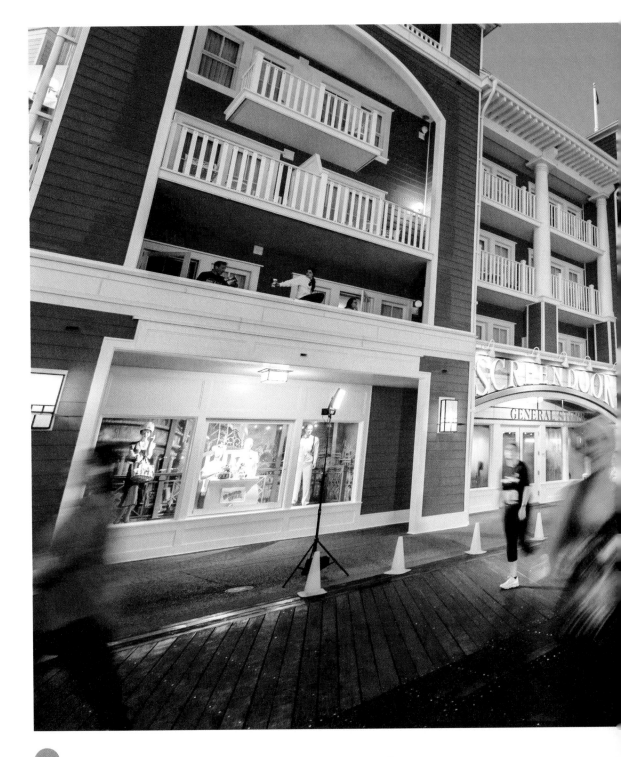

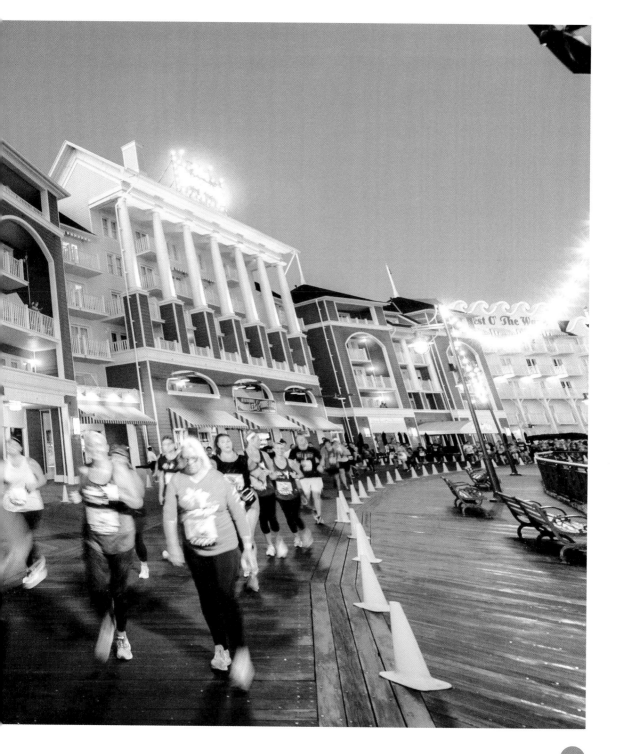

WHERE TO FIND HEALTHY EATS

WALT DISNEY WORLD

BARBECUE

- Flame Tree Barbecue (Animal Kingdom, Discovery Island)

- House of Blues Smokehouse (Disney Springs, West Side)

- The Polite Pig (Disney Springs, Town Center)

- Whispering Canyon Café (Disney's Wilderness Lodge Resort)

BUFFETS

- Biergarten (EPCOT, World Showcase)

- Boma—Flavors of Africa (Disney's Animal Kingdom Lodge)

- Cape May Cafe (Disney's Beach Club Resort)

- Chef Mickey's (Disney's Contemporary Resort)

- Hollywood & Vine (Disney's Hollywood Studios)

- Tusker House (Animal Kingdom, Harambe)

BRUNCH

- Chef Art Smith's Homecomin' (Disney Springs, The Landing; Saturday and Sunday)

- House of Blues (Disney Springs, West Side; Sunday)

- Maria & Enzo's (Disney Springs; Sunday)

- Paddlefish (Disney Springs, The Landing; Sunday)

- Raglan Road (Disney Springs, The Landing; Saturday and Sunday)

- Trail's End (Fort Wilderness; Saturday and Sunday)

INTERNATIONAL EATERIES

- Boma—Flavors of Africa (Disney's Animal Kingdom Lodge)

- Harambe Market (Animal Kingdom, Harambe)

- Jiko—The Cooking Place (Disney's Animal Kingdom Lodge)

- Sanaa (Disney's Animal Kingdom Lodge, Kidani Village)

- Spice Road Table (EPCOT, World Showcase)

- Tangierine Café (EPCOT, World Showcase)

- Tiffins Restaurant (Animal Kingdom, Discovery Island)

- Toledo (Disney's Animal Kingdom Lodge)

- Tusker House (Animal Kingdom, Harambe)

SALADS

- ABC Commissary (Disney's Hollywood Studios)

- Artist's Palette (Disney's Saratoga Springs Resort)

Big River Grill & Brewing Works (Disney's BoardWalk Inn)

Boathouse (Disney Springs, The Landing)

Boma—Flavors of Africa (Disney's Animal Kingdom Lodge)

Chef Art Smith's Homecomin' (Disney Springs, The Landing)

Columbia Harbour House (Magic Kingdom, Liberty Square)

Earl of Sandwich (Disney Springs, Marketplace)

El Mercado de Coronado (Disney's Coronado Springs Resort)

Gasparilla Island Grill (Disney's Grand Floridian Resort & Spa)

Hollywood Brown Derby (Disney's Hollywood Studios)

Il Mulino New York Trattoria (Swan)

Pinocchio Village Haus (Magic Kingdom, Fantasyland)

Plaza Restaurant (Magic Kingdom, Main Street, U.S.A.)

Rainforest Cafe (Animal Kingdom and Disney Springs, Marketplace)

Sunshine Seasons (EPCOT, Future World)

Wolfgang Puck Bar & Grill (Disney Springs, Town Center)

Yak & Yeti (Animal Kingdom, Asia)

SEAFOOD

Ale & Compass Restaurant (Disney's Yacht Club Resort)

Boathouse (Disney Springs, The Landing)

California Grill (Disney's Contemporary Resort)

Cape May Cafe (Disney's Beach Club Resort)

Columbia Harbour House (Magic Kingdom, Liberty Square)

Coral Reef (EPCOT, Future World)

Flying Fish (BoardWalk Inn)

Kimonos (Swan)

Kona Cafe (Disney's Polynesian Village Resort)

Monsieur Paul (EPCOT, World Showcase)

Narcoossee's (Disney's Grand Floridian Resort & Spa)

Paddlefish (Disney Springs, The Landing)

Sebastian's Bistro (Disney's Caribbean Beach Resort)

Todd English's bluezoo (Dolphin)

Tokyo Dining (EPCOT, World Showcase)

Victoria & Albert's (Disney's Grand Floridian Resort & Spa)

SOLO DINERS

- Boathouse (Disney Springs, The Landing)

- Cítricos Lounge (Disney's Grand Floridian Resort & Spa)

- Crew's Cup (Disney's Yacht Club Resort)

- Enzo's Hideaway (Disney Springs, The Landing)

- Flying Fish (Disney's BoardWalk Inn)

- Il Mulino New York Trattoria (Swan)

- Jiko—The Cooking Place Lounge (Disney's Animal Kingdom Lodge)

- Narcoossee's Lounge (Disney's Grand Floridian Resort & Spa)

- Nomad Lounge (Disney's Animal Kingdom, Discovery Island)

- Paddlefish (Disney Springs, The Landing)

- Raglan Road (Disney Springs, The Landing)

- Tune-In Lounge (Disney's Hollywood Studios)

- Wine Bar George (Disney Springs, The Landing)

SUSHI

- Benihana Steakhouse and Sushi (Hilton Orlando Lake Buena Vista hotel)

- California Grill (Disney's Contemporary Resort)

- Kabuki Cafe (EPCOT, World Showcase)

- Katsura Grill (EPCOT, World Showcase)

- Kimonos (Swan)

- Kona Cafe (Disney's Polynesian Village Resort)

- Kona Island (after 5:00 p.m.; Disney's Polynesian Village Resort)

- Morimoto Asia (Disney Springs, The Landing)

- Splitsville (Disney Springs, West Side)

- Tokyo Dining (EPCOT, World Showcase)

PLANT-BASED

- Boma—Flavors of Africa (Disney's Animal Kingdom Lodge)

- Columbia Harbour House (Magic Kingdom, Liberty Square)

- Cosmic Ray's Starlight Café (Magic Kingdom, Tomorrowland)

- Everything Pop! (Disney's Pop Century Resort)

- Food Courts (All-Star Resorts)

- Jiko—The Cooking Place (Animal Kingdom Lodge)

- La Hacienda de San Angel (EPCOT, World Showcase)

- Les Halles Boulangerie Patisserie (EPCOT, World Showcase)

- Mama Melrose's Ristorante Italiano (Disney's Hollywood Studios)

- Pinocchio Village Haus (Magic Kingdom, Fantasyland)

- Pizzafari (Animal Kingdom, Discovery Island)

- PizzeRizzo (Disney's Hollywood Studios)

- Rainforest Cafe (Animal Kingdom and Disney Springs, Marketplace)

- Sanaa (Disney's Animal Kingdom Lodge, Kidani Village)

- Sunset Ranch Market (Disney's Hollywood Studios)

- Sunshine Seasons (EPCOT, Future World)

- Teppan Edo (EPCOT, World Showcase)

- Tony's Town Square (Magic Kingdom, Main Street, U.S.A.)

- Tusker House (Animal Kingdom, Harambe)

- Tutto Italia (EPCOT, World Showcase)

- Via Napoli (EPCOT, World Showcase)

DISNEYLAND

BUFFET

- Goofy's Kitchen (Disneyland Hotel)

- Storytellers Café (Disney's Grand Californian Hotel & Spa)

- Plaza Inn (Disneyland Park, Main Street, U.S.A.)

BRUNCH

- Lamplight Lounge (Disney California Adventure Park, Pixar Pier)

- Storytellers Café (Disney's Grand Californian Hotel & Spa)

PLANT-BASED

- Ballast Point Brewing Co. (Downtown Disney District)

- Boardwalk Pizza and Pasta (Disney California Adventure Park, Paradise Gardens Park)

- Earl of Sandwich (Downtown Disney District)

- GCH Craftsman Grill (Disney's Grand Californian Hotel & Spa)

- Lamplight Lounge (Disney California Adventure Park, Pixar Pier)

- Rancho del Zocalo (Disneyland Park, Frontierland)

- Red Rose Taverne (Disneyland Park, Fantasyland)

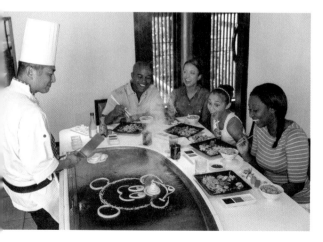

ABOUT THE AUTHORS

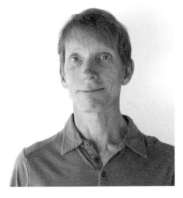

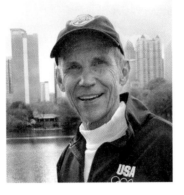

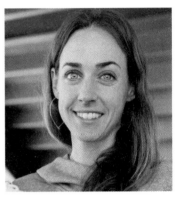

SCOTT DOUGLAS (main text) is a contributing writer for *Runner's World*, and the author or coauthor of several books, including two *New York Times* best sellers. Among his books are *Running Is My Therapy*, *Meb for Mortals*, *Advanced Marathoning*, and *The Athlete's Guide to CBD*. A lifelong runner who has put in more than 100,000 miles, Scott lives in South Portland, Maine.

JEFF GALLOWAY (foreword and select sidebars) is the official runDisney coach and the inventor of the Galloway Run-Walk-Run Method. Hundreds of thousands of runners have used his training programs to complete marathons and half marathons—and have fun while doing so. Jeff's books include *The Run-Walk-Run Method*, *Running Until You're 100*, *Marathon: You Can Do It*, and *Mental Training for Runners*. A member of the 1972 U.S. Olympic team, Jeff lives in Atlanta.

MOLLY HUDDLE (select sidebars) is a two-time Olympian who holds the American records for 10,000 meters and the half marathon. She has won more than twenty-five U.S. titles. Molly is the cocreator and cohost of the *Keeping-Track* podcast. She lives in Providence, Rhode Island.

ACKNOWLEDGMENTS

I have to start by thanking my incredible team and partners who make coming to work and putting on runDisney events a true joy. I am humbled and honored to work with the best of the best. Thank you to Jennifer Levesque and the entire team at Disney Publishing. Thanks to Scott Douglas for writing this book, capturing all of the things that make runDisney races so magical, and putting it into words. A special thanks to Olympians Jeff Galloway and Molly Huddle for adding their insight and experience in endurance running. And, finally, thank you to the loyal and dedicated runDisney fans. Your love and passion for runDisney is a constant source of inspiration for us.

—Faron D. Kelley, runDisney

Thanks to this book's editor, Jennifer Levesque, for bringing me on board this project, and for her patience, support, and guidance throughout the writing and editing process. Thanks to Audra Wason, Kimberly Keller, Heidi Pickert, and Tina Trybus at runDisney, as well as Jon Hughes and Tom Ward for their insider takes on runDisney history and courses. Finally, I'm honored to have as my coauthors Olympians Jeff Galloway and Molly Huddle.

—Scott Douglas

PLAN A MAGICAL RUNCATION WITH THE ONLY OFFICIAL GUIDES TO THE DISNEY PARKS AND RESORTS!

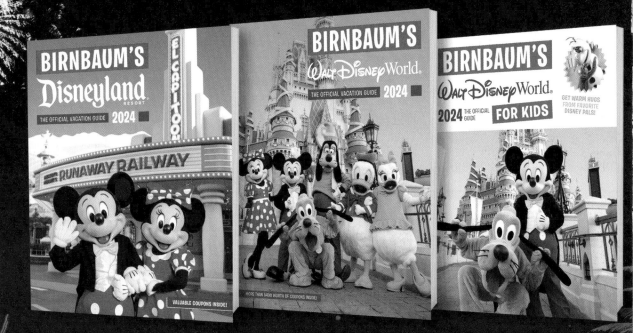

Featuring expert advice and reviews, the most up to date information, coupons, and more!

AVAILABLE WHEREVER BOOKS ARE SOLD.